THE LOWDOWN ON

GOING
DOWN

Also by Marcy Michaels
with Marie DeSalle

Blow Him Away

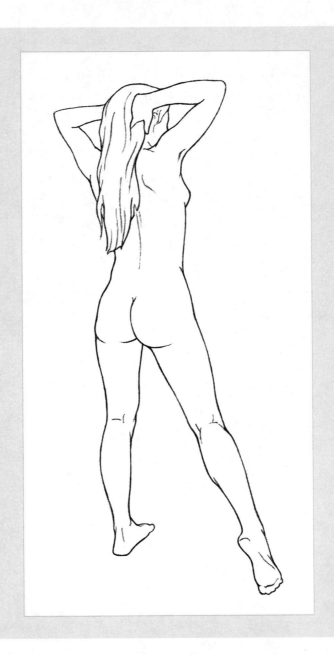

THE LOWDOWN ON

GOING DOWN

HOW TO GIVE HER

MIND-BLOWING ORAL SEX

MARCY MICHAELS

with Marie DeSalle

BROADWAY BOOKS NEW YORK

BROADWAY

DISCLAIMER: The instructions and advice in this book are in no way intended as a substitute for medical counseling. We advise the reader to consult with his/her doctor before beginning this or any other exercise regimen. The author and the publisher disclaim any liability or loss, personal or otherwise, resulting from the exercises in this book.

Broadway Books titles may be purchased for business or promotional use or for special sales. For information, please write to: Special Markets Department, Random House, Inc., 1745 Broadway, New York, NY 10019.

PRINTED IN THE UNITED STATES OF AMERICA

BROADWAY BOOKS and its logo, a letter B bisected on the diagonal, are trademarks of Random House, Inc.

Visit our website at www.broadwaybooks.com

First edition published 2005

Book design by JoAnne Metsch

Library of Congress Cataloging-in-Publication Data

Michaels, Marcy.
    The lowdown on going down / Marcy Michaels with Marie DeSalle.—1st ed.
        p. cm.
    Includes bibliographical references.
    1. Sex instruction for men. 2. Oral sex. 3. Female orgasm. I. DeSalle, Marie. II. Title.

HQ36.M53 2005
613.9'6—dc22

2004050266

ISBN 0-7679-1657-3

5 7 9 10 8 6 4

That man that hath a tongue, I say, is no man,
If with his tongue he cannot win a woman.

—WILLIAM SHAKESPEARE,
The Two Gentlemen of Verona, Act 3

CONTENTS

On the Orgasm That Inspired This Book

T SOME POINT, almost everyone asks me how I first made the connection between speech therapy and oral sex. Did it just hit me one day? Was it in a dream? Did one of my patients clue me into the "side benefits" of my therapy? The answer requires a little background information.

My history and upbringing were far from sexually liberated. I grew up thinking that a woman's place was in the home, and more in the kitchen than the bedroom. To top that off, I married my first boyfriend. If you had asked me where my G-spot was, I might have pointed somewhere near my knee. "Naïve" doesn't begin to convey how oblivious I was to the various parts of my body and their ability to generate sensual pleasure. The ever-blossoming sexual revolution that swept across the nation barely touched me, incubated as I was in a thankless marriage on the Upper East Side of Manhattan with no career of my own, and not a single sex toy to my name. Inexplicably (I thought) unhappy, I finally went to see a psychiatrist. As I sat in his deceptively nondescript office, he concluded that my problems stemmed from a lack of sexual experience. I had only been with one person, he reasoned, how could I know what I wanted? Taken aback by his prescription—"have sex with new partners as soon as possible"—I went out in search of a less wanton opinion.

Sexual liberation must have been going around that year, because psychiatrists numbers two, three, and four all gave me the same homework: take your sexuality into your own hands. Driven to the edge of despair by my unfulfilling marriage, I desperately, wildly, did just that—I took my sexuality into my own hands, and the rest of my life came with it. I divorced my husband, started my career as a speech pathologist, and got busy on the New York dating scene.

I was a woman on a mission. Having always been interested in helping others and the power of speech, I decided to pursue an advanced degree in speech pathology. By day I went to my speech classes, and by night I broke loose on the grand ole isle of Manhattan. Professionally, I was studying with some of the most enlightened people in my field. Personally, I was dating a sampling of the best lovers New York had to offer. I was thoroughly enjoying myself in both of these new worlds. The oral sex discovery resulted from an unlikely intersection of the two.

One day, on a trip to Atlantic City, I met a tall, pleasant fellow who took me around for the day. By that time, I was a little jaded. I had been dating for years by then, and thought I had seen everything. It was a fairly standard date—that is, until he gave me a good-night kiss that made my knees buckle and my stomach flip. My mouth, partially lost in his, seemed to be transcending into new realms, while my legs became heavy and sank toward the boardwalk. Sparks were sent flying all over my body, and an electrical current seemed to be running through my veins. Before long, we were inside my room at the hotel, and I was experiencing all-over body orgasms that challenged my definition of an orgasm as something with a beginning and an end.

And he did it all night long without a gasp, a hesitation, or a slackening of energy.

Now this guy wasn't unusually charming or attractive. While his personality was fine and friendly, it was nothing to write home about, and his anatomy was entirely average. His tongue and mouth alone were responsible for my pleasure-fest, and immediately advanced him to the top of my list. So what transformed this mere mortal into an oral superman? Have you guessed yet? Of all things, Supermouth was trained as a *speech therapist*. I returned to my speech pathology classes in New York with a newfound enthusiasm.

This book is dedicated to sharing the secrets I learned in my years practicing speech therapy. They will help you gain a new mastery over your lips and tongue, enabling you to send shivers up your lover's spine on command. To make sure you get the most out of these techniques, I've included a handy, step-by-step guide to giving your lucky lady the best oral sex of her life.

So let's get you started.

BEFORE WE BEGIN: A NOTE ON SAFETY

The techniques set forth in this book are largely intended for the comparatively safe setting of a monogamous, long-term relationship. Of course, they can be practiced on anyone, at any time, but they are meant to be experienced with someone you know well and trust. Though oral sex has been proven to be less likely to transmit HIV and other STDs than unprotected intercourse, the possibility still exists. Furthermore, if your partner has a bacterial STD, it is possible to contract it in your mouth or throat, or anywhere you have mucous membranes (including your nose). Keep in mind that the person performing these activities—doing the licking, sucking, or taking fluids into their mouth—is much more at risk than the person being licked, sucked, and generating the fluids. If you're getting intimate with someone you don't know very well, make sure you protect yourself with a condom or dental dam.

There are as many different kinds of protection available today as there are positions in the *Kama Sutra*, and some of them are designed to add to the fun with flavoring and ribs. Before things get hot and heavy, find the products best suited to your needs that will allow you to be safe while exploring and expanding your sexual boundaries. Information on this topic abounds on the Internet (the Society for Human Sexuality at www.sexuality.org is a good starting place) and can also be found in numerous publications. Please do whatever is safest for you, so that you can delve into your sexual experiences with a truly carefree spirit.

Introduction

TO SUCK OR NOT TO SUCK: THAT IS THE QUESTION

THIS GUIDE IS based on the premise that oral sex can—and should—be outrageously fantastic *every time*. The poor quality of much oral sex being performed today can be baffling at first, but it becomes more understandable when one considers the factors involved. There are a plethora of psychological and social reasons that the tongue tickle hasn't been cultivated as a talent, but more often than not, a fatally simple want of skill and knowledge is to blame. This guide addresses both situations, but is mostly devoted to the latter.

When you engage in oral sex, you're taking the most delicate, vulnerable part of your lover's body—their genitals—and placing them between the most potentially vicious, animalistic part of yours—your teeth. The teeth are situated in the mouth to gnash, process food, and ward off harm. It's a wonderfully human quirk that we use this part of our body to give pleasure. Ironically, this distinctively human trait has been characterized by previous generations as dirty and uncivilized.

I don't need to argue here about the importance of great sex to the health of a romantic relationship. We've all seen TV shows and movies that portray sex and passion as über-racy, with bodies writhing in satin sheets under perfectly dimmed lighting, as if little elves had benevolently prepped the room for a one-two-three orgasm. But if sex and romance are overvalued, oral sex is all too frequently undervalued in the media and culture at large.

Still occasionally stigmatized as "dirtier" than straight-up sex, the power of oral sex for sustaining and deepening a romantic relationship often gets overlooked. Sharing pleasure, as in intercourse, and *giving* pleasure have very different effects on a relationship, simply because they have very different effects on your partner. Being able to *give* pleasure to your partner, unselfishly and lovingly, can be very important and plays a different role in your interpersonal dynamic. Oral sex is special in that it makes the other person feel cared for, tended to, and looked after. If actions speak louder than words, oral sex is like speaking through a megaphone when you tell your partner that you like and enjoy them.

Yet somehow, despite all this being so, most people don't perform oral sex as well as they could. In fact, most people sort of suck at oral sex. But it doesn't have to stay this way—we can choose to raise the status quo.

Oral sex must be performed properly to be effective and enjoyable. Unless your mouth is strong and controlled, there's a limit to how much pleasure you'll be capable of giving your lover. For instance, there's a special way of elevating the clitoris through the suction of the lips, and then holding this position and stimulating it with a circular motion of the tongue that reliably drives women to ecstasy (this technique is illustrated on page 103). But a normal person frankly doesn't have enough jaw control—not to mention lip strength and fine manipulation—to pull it off. Most people can't even tie a cherry stem in their mouth.

Drawing on my experiences with patients, I can tell you that an average person trying to perform the move just mentioned would have a very high likelihood of slackening their jaw control while they tried to keep up the muscular action of the tongue, leading the jaw to close in what could be a *very* painful little mishap. The most pleasurable moves require a level of expertise that most of us simply don't have. When it comes to oral sex, we need more than a list of good ideas, no matter how tantalizing those might be.

"My boyfriend seems confused," a friend once told me, "he thinks that oral sex is just a way to make it wet down there so that we can have intercourse." Another problem with this "significant, beautiful" human act is that few people are willing to give oral sex its due. When it comes time to go down, some people flat-out avoid it, while others treat it like a chore. But in terms of sexual satisfaction, this is outright pleasure sabotage, given that many people view oral sex as actually *more* pleasurable than intercourse. (A whopping 92 percent of "career women" surveyed prefer it to any other sex act.)* It's time to face it, folks: *oral sex may be your most powerful sexual tool.*

Because your partner can lay back and focus all of their attention on the sensations you're providing, oral sex is a highly memorable sex act. So, when things have been heating up, and it's time to dive between

---

* Samuel S. Janus, Ph.D., and Cynthia L. Janus, Ph.D. *The Janus Report on Sexual Behavior* (New York: John Wiley and Sons, 1993).

the sheets (or unzip in the middle of the living room, as you prefer), before you perform oral sex, ask yourself: How do I want to be remembered? As someone who can give pleasure generously, or a skimp who's trying to hurry things along? To have your lover beating down your door for years to come, you need to give them more than one "oh-my-god-oh-my-god-oh-my-god" sensation—you need to be able to exploit the vast diversity of feelings that can be unlocked with just a tiny bit of muscular mastery, the oohs and aahs that are the bread and butter of great oral sex.

You may think you know everything you need to about oral sex, and that there's nothing a guide could tell you that you can't figure out for yourself. Vis-à-vis most guides out there, you're right. The majority of books about sex either recycle old material, or in their hunt for novelty come up with positions more suited for Gumby and Pokey than for you and your partner. But few of them prescribe the single ingredient that is widely needed: tongue and lip exercises.

Here you have the fruits of an entire field of study, developed by experts and researchers for more than a hundred years, recontextualized and applied to oral sex for the first time. And it's only logical: Out of all of the available specialists, wouldn't you want a doctor of the mouth to help you or your partner perform oral sex?

In my practice as a speech pathologist, I've seen that what most people need is basic training. They need to strengthen and energize their mouths, lips, and throats so that they can perform *any* and *all* techniques with absolute comfort. Unless you're strong at your base, sophisticated techniques will never help you. In fact, students of sexual technique can (and have) hurt themselves or their partner while trying out new things. Giving your partner the best oral sex of her life isn't going to happen with just a couple of new techniques. You have to establish your muscular strength, refine your control, and *then* you can employ the moan-making, sheet-ripping, multiple orgasm–generating techniques.

WHY SPEECH THERAPY IS OLYMPIC TRAINING FOR ORAL SEX

Thirty years ago, when I started practicing speech therapy, I would have laughed at the idea of me—or anyone else in my industry—writing an oral sex guide. Speech therapy belongs with dentists, orthodontists, and speech analysts, not Dr. Ruth, sex therapy, and dental dams . . . right? While it's perfectly true that most branches of speech therapy have nothing to do with oral sex, and while there may be a practitioner or two out there who's never even *had* oral sex, speech therapy nonetheless has designed techniques that will blow your partner's socks off (if they're still on). So don't go swinging the gavel too soon. You can't judge a field of study by its unerotic exterior. The quality of oral sex increases so rapidly when these techniques are applied that they almost seem better for sex than they are for speech.

But you can't chalk up these oral sex results to common speech therapy. Practiced at its most general, the entire field couldn't help you get a single sigh out of your lover. Except perhaps from boredom. Lots of speech therapy involves repeating monosyllables from a droning tape with a monitoring instructor. Great way to spend the afternoon, right? I didn't think so, either. In addition to being a speech pathologist, I was also trained as a myofunctional (literally "muscle-function") therapist. Myofunctional therapy is the speech specialization that most directly applies to oral sex. In myofunctional therapy, muscles are gods: they can push and pull teeth around at their whim. They can bring a bone out of alignment, or they can bring one into alignment. It all depends on how the muscle has been trained to interact with other bodily systems. In the fight between muscle and bone (and these fights are taking place all over your body), muscles always win. They have an agency that no other part of the body can lay claim to. There's reason people say they were "muscled" into doing something (although being "boned" has pretty straightforward connotations of its own).

You may think that your tongue is a soft, pink love muscle that simply rests in your mouth until you need it to chew or speak or get sexy. But it's the most powerful muscle in your body in terms of exerting force, and as any speech therapist can tell you, that little sucker is exerting force all day long. The tongue exerts a minimum of six (and a maximum of eight) pounds of pressure in your mouth *each* time you swallow. The average individual swallows one thousand times in a twenty-four-hour cycle. You don't need to be a math wiz to figure out that that's a *lot* of pressure—at least six thousand pounds a day—to be exerting anywhere in your body. And it's more than enough to alter the structure of your mouth and the placement of your teeth significantly.

There is a right way and a wrong way to place your tongue in your mouth. If we could feel just a little more of the six thousand pounds of pressure our tongues exert every day, most people would figure out how to place their tongues correctly as a matter of urgency. There's a part of the mouth that's designed to withstand the pressure of the tongue—the hard palate on the roof—but most people never use it. Instead, they rest their tongues between their teeth, in the bottom of their jaw, or even worse, against the backs of the top teeth. Over time, placing the tongue in each of these spots *weakens* the tongue and surrounding muscles. As you read this paragraph, where is your tongue in your mouth? If it's anywhere other than resting on the roof of your mouth behind (but not touching) the top row of teeth, your oral sex ability is being compromised. Try this experiment: read the rest of this book with the tip of your tongue *always* pressing against the hard palate on the roof of your mouth, without touching your teeth. Have it be the first thing you do when you open this book. (For an illustration of where you should place it, turn to page 30.)

A poorly placed tongue impairs any and all uses of the tongue and mouth. Most people don't know that this is an issue—while performing oral sex, they might just think that it's natural to feel strained, get lockjaw, or have a gag reflex. While kissing, they might think that it's equally normal to feel like they can't get their lips in the right spot. But all of these (and snoring!) are symptoms of a misplaced tongue.

Aside from these effects, the placement of these incremental bursts of pressure changes the shape of your jaw and the placement of your teeth; determines how free your tongue is to move in, out, and around your mouth; and influences how much energy it has. You probably didn't know that every time you swallow, you're either helping or hurting your greatest oral sex asset. You probably didn't even *want* to know that. But if you do want to give mind-blowing, satisfying, remembered-with-a-grin oral sex each and every time (and if you want to have fun doing it), you're gonna have to accept a few Tongue Realities.

Tongue Reality 1: Your tongue does not like it when you smoke. I know, I know, it's sexy (sort of) and it can be a way to bond with Mr. or Ms. Unapproachable Smoker, but the fact is that smoking isn't good for your tongue. A smoker's tongue tends to be lazy and lifeless, bulbous and placid. Your tongue needs to be an energetic, frontward, stand-up soldier, not a limp pile of mess hall meat. Not to mention, smoking is flat-out bad for you, so it's not like you would be getting rid of a productive pastime.

Tongue Reality 2: Your tongue needs exercise, too. You may think that your tongue gets a fine workout by eating and talking and frenching cuties, but usually quite the opposite is happening. Since most people don't even know the right position for their tongue, these activities actually weaken it by reinforcing bad habits. If you want a tongue that can lead wild excursions into intensely sensual experiences, you have to give it specific, controlled exercises. In chapter 4, you'll find some of the exercises to jump-start basic training for your tongue.

Tongue Reality 3: You don't know your tongue. Maybe you're lucky enough to have already gone to speech therapy (though you might not have recognized this as luck at the time). Or maybe you were even luckier and inherently assumed correct tongue positioning. But it's highly unlikely: out of more than ten thousand patients I've seen, not a single one walked into my office with their tongue correctly placed. Most of them didn't even know that there *was* a correct position for the tongue. But take heart—tongues are easy to get to know. They have simple needs that are easily satisfied. And you and your partner are going to get a lot out of this new acquaintance. Speaking of which, there's a list of side benefits to these exercises that could lure the biggest couch potatoes on the planet to open their mouths and exercise their love tool:

You'll Feel Better
Much of your body's tension goes into the face, neck, and shoulders and stays there. We grind our teeth. We can't get our sinuses unclogged. We get short of breath sooner than we should, not from ex-

ertion but from not breathing properly. All these symptoms can be exercised away.

You'll Look Better

With your jaw muscles balanced, your tongue in the right place, and your swallowing patterns corrected, your face in repose will be at its most symmetrical and unstressed, so your features can appear to their best advantage. When you smile, talk, sing, or make love, you won't be contorted, look tense, or appear worried, because your face will stop storing muscular tension—you'll be radiating charm instead of strain.

You'll Sound Better

Your voice will have a wonderful resonance, both richer and rounder than you've probably ever heard it. It will be sexier, more commanding. When you open your mouth to speak, your voice will have more tonal assurance, making people more likely to want to listen and respond to you.

Furthermore, if you snore (or if you're one of the thousands of unwitting youngsters who will begin snoring in the next twenty years), performing these exercises and keeping your tongue correctly positioned will eliminate the possibility of a single little snore—or even a midnight chortle—ever escaping your lips. When the tongue is positioned correctly, your mouth is physiologically incapable of snoring.

You'll Know More

You'll be able to check out a great deal about a prospective lover in advance—by the time you've completed the exercises in this book, a quick tongue reading and an assessment of face, mouth, and voice will tell you all that you need to know about a potential oral sex partner.

Now that you are familiar with these basic notions, it's time to start preparing you to deliver lifelong ecstasy. Many oral sex lovers are inadvertently lopsided—either they have lots of enthusiasm and lack the required skills, or they have some know-how but no panache. The following chapters are dedicated to making sure that you're a well-rounded lover.

I

Even Tiger Woods Has to Practice:
Preparing Yourself to Find (and Swing)
Your Partner of Choice

> If sex is such a natural phenomenon, how come
> there are so many books on how to?
> —BETTE MIDLER

I T WOULD BE a cause for celebration if we were born with the natural and intuitive set of sexual skills that we all pretend we have. Without stating it outright, our culture—via our parents, the media, and our peers—implies that sex and sexual skills should come naturally, with all but the most advanced techniques being somehow instinctive. You'd never expect someone to hit a perfect tennis serve without lessons and practice or to play a beautiful sonata on an instrument they've only touched a couple of times, yet somehow, most of us come to maturity with the expectation that sexual skills will magically develop in the presence of our naked lover, that this lover will likewise experience a spontaneous onset of spectacular proficiency, and that it will all unfurl as smoothly as a movie montage.

Where do real-life Don Juans get their savoir faire? There's only one way: practice, practice, practice. Some people try to pick up tips from their friends, but while you may have a friend or two with information to spare, you're probably dealing with what literary critics calls an "unreliable narrator." (I personally stopped trusting the sexual knowledge of my peers when they asked me if my cherry had been popped, but could not specify what this "cherry" was, nor exactly where it was located.)

Real sex is awkward. The fact is, if you expect great sex to come naturally, you're in big trouble, and your partner is in even bigger trouble. Giving great oral sex is dependent upon being truly comfortable with the act, "in good times and in bad." Real sex with live people is tricky—it smells, it squeaks, it gets stuck on some things and rams too quickly into others. People get injured physically (especially in the shower) and emotionally (especially in affairs), and on the whole, doing it probably causes about as many problems as pleasures. This doesn't mean that you should stop, in fact most of us should be having more sex rather than less. But it does indicate that we have a lot of false expectations surrounding sex, and these expectations take a lot of the fun out of sex without our even knowing it.

ACCEPTING THESE REALITIES WILL MAKE YOU A BETTER LOVER

Sexual Skill Doesn't Come Naturally

Sure, the impulse to have sex is "natural," and the heat of passion is sure to lend a little on-the-spot inspiration, but sexual skill must be learned and practiced like anything else.

"If girls are made of sugar and spice, why do they taste like tuna fish?"
Genitals have a naturally pungent odor and taste. Some people love it, others don't. But you're in denial if you're surprised by it. If this is a concern for you, just take a bath or shower with your partner, instead of trying to skirt oral sex, or pretending to be comfortable going down when you're not. If you forge ahead anyway, your partner will sense your repressed discomfort, and the effort to conceal your true feelings will take the zest out of your performance. Barring a bath, be aware that a vagina will taste and smell very differently after it is stimulated enough to create the body's natural lubricants, which have an addictively delicious flavor. A little foreplay and hand action can change the menu entirely.

A Funny Thing Happened on the Way to the Orgasm

What's the matter? Labia got yer tongue? Whether it's that funny slurping noise, a penis that veers to the right like it's catching a curve ball, or a pubic hair in your eye, unexpected things are bound to happen during sex. Who can say what they will be? One woman I know started laughing while her guy was coming in her mouth, and it ended up dribbling out of her nose. Things like this are a natural part of an active sex life, so you might as well expect them and make sure to bring your sense of humor with you to the bedroom. Taking sex too seriously is a sure passion-killer.

Genitals Look Funny

Believe it or not, the overall quality of oral sex is still being compromised by people's shame and fear of genitalia. The people giving oral sex are afraid to stare too much, because they don't want to make their partner feel uncomfortable, while their partner can barely even relax and enjoy themselves because they're so freaked out by someone sniffing around down there. Shocking as it is, this is occurring in the twenty-first century, and it's compromising the quality of oral sex. To overcome any vestiges of genital-fear, take a moment with your partner to really look at her genitals. Tell her why you want to do it, and make sure that she feels comfortable with it first. Then look—really *look*—at all the different parts, and acknowledge that these are what you have to work with. This exercise is worth it: an anatomically complete understanding of your partner's genitals will assure your subconscious that there is nothing "bad" or "dirty" or "scary" lurking in there anywhere.

"That was great. Really, it was . . ."

Most likely, no one's told you the truth about your sexual skills. The fact is, women fake orgasms pretty regularly, and it's a rare lover who openly communicates what they do or don't like, because they're trying to be nice. But withholding feedback is extremely counterproductive with regards to sex. The way people communicate about sex isn't even worthy of the term "miscommunication," because not only does withholding feedback send the wrong information (that you like something you don't or dislike something you do like), it actively obstructs future communication about sex. We're lucky consultants can't be called into the bedroom, because most people would be fired. The result? Very few men and women have been given enough feedback to develop a repertoire that works. And it's a damned shame. Since they haven't built up the strength and precision of their lips and tongue through a history of feedback and refinement, they develop a repertoire based on second-rate skills that every sexual partner is subjected to. As a loving pet-owner thinks their cat or dog is absolutely unique, everyone—and I mean *everyone*—thinks they have great sexual skills. Meanwhile, most people report more than a few instances of less-than-satisfying sex every year. You do the math.

You don't have to pass out a Comments and Suggestions card afterward, but you do need to elicit your partner's feedback. A whispered "Do you like that?" during oral sex will produce more honest feedback than a "Was that good for you?" after she's already decided that she just wants to be friends.

It's Not Just About the Orgasm

You don't have to make your partner come to have great oral sex. Great oral lovers are not orgasm-making machines, and if you treat oral sex this way you're not going to enjoy it—and neither will your partner. Aside from straining yourself, your orgasm fixation will actually distract you from any subtle signs or signals given by your lover. You don't have to frantically chase orgasms through the thickets of your lover's genitals. The orgasm will come to you. Straining and stressing about how long it's taking your partner to come wards off a real orgasm like a snake scares a mare, so it's better to just let go of this expectation and enjoy yourself. Experiment and play—"the light touch," as it's sometimes called—will inevitably create more pleasure for your partner than strain or stress.

People who perform poorly at oral sex are usually hung up on one or all of these basic issues. But there's another, related set of issues that are a little more serious and must be addressed for you to get the most out of giving—and getting—oral sex.

2

When Your Mind Spoils Your Head:
What Wrecks Oral Sex

NO MATTER HOW much you might try to convince yourself that you are a sexual cavalier and not a vulnerable human being, sex is an intimate act. It almost always brings up somebody's emotions. Oral sex is in some ways even more intimate. There's a Chinese proverb that says if you save a person's life, they're yours forever. That's fine and well, but hair-pulling, moan-making, nail-sinking oral sex breeds its own strain of attachment, and it can be pretty fierce.

Partially because of the intense feelings of vulnerability it can provoke, some people have a very hard time opening themselves up to receiving oral sex. At the thought of someone else fully exploring their genitals and witnessing their states of uncontrolled ecstasy, some people begin to drool, while others snap closed like a clam. (Personally, I drool.) Control issues (*after all, what might that other person do down there? Will they try to stick something weird in my [insert most feared orifice here] or do something else that I'm not prepared for?*), self-doubt (*Do I smell down there? What if I have to fart? What if I didn't wipe well the last time I . . . you know . . ?*), and a negative body-image (*Are they noticing my love-handles/cellulite/ass hairs or whatever aspect of my body I despair over?*), as well as a plethora of other issues can take the fun out of oral sex faster than you can say the word "orgasm." And that's just on the receiving end!

On the giving end, performance anxiety and fear of being judged are chief among the pleasure killers. *"What if they don't like what I'm doing?" "What if I get tired and need to stop before they've had an orgasm?" "What if I can't bring them to orgasm?"* And for those who are hip to all the orgasm-faking going on: *"What if they're just pretending to like it?"* You may be surprised just how many people let thoughts like these crash their oral sex party.

While there is no magic potion to remove these inhibitions (other than drugs and alcohol, which are *not* long-term solutions!), there are some steps, before, during, and after your rendezvous that can help you to better relax and enjoy yourself. Being comfortable and happy make almost anything you do better, and this goes double for oral sex. In order to devote yourself fully to giving and receiving pleasure, you need to be as deep in the pleasure groove as you can get.

GETTING READY TO RUMBLE:
A DATING GUIDE FOR FABULOUS ORAL LOVE

For those of you who are perfectly comfortable with your body, have no trouble relaxing and getting down to business, and are 100 percent ready for action, skip this bit and go straight to chapter 3. For those of you who have been single for a while, tend to fumble with sexual tension, or simply feel that you could be better at relaxing and enjoying the ride, here's some information on how to prepare your *entire* being for oral sex.

Before going out with a sexual partner or soon-to-be sexual partner, most people spend time squinting in the mirror and picking out their most flattering clothes. Paying a little extra attention to your appearance and hygiene before a date is a natural inclination—and should be de rigueur if you're hoping for future dates—but the buck rarely stops there. All over the country, people go tearing through their closets looking for the "right" outfit, wrestling into one sweater just to run to the mirror and frown. "You're fat," the mirror says back, "and I'm not granting you any wishes." Noticing a new pimple or wrinkle just before a date has furrowed countless brows. "This big, ugly pimple next to my mouth looks *awful*—they'll probably think I have herpes! Maybe I should just cancel." These thoughts and feelings aren't restricted to ephemera—our more substantial physical "flaws" provoke even more nerve-racking thoughts. "My pubic hair is turning silver," an older friend confided in me, "and I don't know what's more painful: their facial expression when my underwear comes off, or plucking the damned things."

Fretting seems harmless, but how are you going to get comfortable and enjoy what your body can do if you've spent all the time before your date chastising it? The seeming innocuousness of predate fretting is only skin-deep: it has very real consequences for sex and physical pleasure.

Shower Power

Being clean and sweet-smelling is a considerate gesture that says to your partner "I want you to enjoy contact with my body," and it can boost your self-confidence. But criticizing your body on *any* level will impede your oral sex performance, because how you feel about your own body will be played out in how you react to your lover's. It can also distract you from your partner's subtle signals, and delay your own orgasms. Is being zitless and well-dressed worth it? Is *anything*? Of course, you should look nice for your date—but obsessive thoughts have a momentum of their own and cannot be cast off as easily as clothing.

Consider limiting your preening time to around fifteen minutes— just enough time to cover the basics, not enough to nitpick. Use the rest of the time to prepare yourself psychologically to have fun and relax.

The Two Big Basics

These are very simple ideas, but disregarded by one and all. First, wear comfortable clothes. Not quite the jeans with holes and your favorite tattered sweater, but make it a rule to avoid tight or restricting clothes, and clothes that are out of character for you. If you don't look like yourself, you won't act like yourself. (Also, it's not a bad idea to save the tight jeans and fancy shirts for a time when you may need the kinkiness.)

Second, use the time before your date to *relax* and *unwind*. If going on your date straight from work, take a walk around the block just to absorb the atmosphere of the neighborhood, or treat yourself to something that will loosen you up—maybe it's listening to music, getting a beer, or going in a pet store and watching puppies tussle. Whatever it is, it needs to relax you. For more serious stress cases, it may take a ten-minute massage or short workout. No matter what your stress level is, though, there's one cure-all: breathing. The breathing exercises outlined in chapter 7 are among the best stress antidotes around. They cost nothing, take little time, and relax you utterly. But if you want to be giving off your most sexual vibes, there are some specific activities that will send sparks flying on contact.

If you don't have time to relax and unwind before a date, simply pop into the bathroom and look at yourself in the mirror. Do you like yourself? If you don't get a resounding, "Hell yeah, I'm awesome!" keep looking at yourself and just say it out loud: "I like me." Say it until you start to mean it, and then you can go rock the world. Feeling good about yourself makes everything you do better.

THE RECEIVING END

This is supposed to be more fun than a roller coaster,
but I feel like I'm still waiting in line . . .

While the majority of this guide is devoted to *giving* oral sex, its raison d'être is to improve the quality of oral sex everywhere, for everyone. With this objective in mind, a little space is devoted here to people who expect to enjoy oral sex, but who, when the time comes, feel uncomfortable or disengaged. If you're already an oral-sex hound, feel free to skip the rest of this chapter and move on to the next. But if you've had some disappointments, stick around.

The Distraction Reaction
All you can think about is what you have to do tomorrow/some overdue project/an obligation, concern, or care of any kind.

This one comes first, because even if you have never experienced this problem, enough months of sharing a bed will bring it along. You don't have to have attention deficit disorder for your mind to wander to all kinds of unrelated subjects—and people—during sex. Oral sex is a particularly likely arena for this because, if you're the recipient, your participation is (usually) not required, and your mental attention even less so. Lots of people are disturbed by their wandering minds, because it seems to indicate a problem in the relationship. But this is usually not the case.

If you notice your thoughts repeatedly turning to the same obligation, concern, or care, take a deep breath first (always rule number one), and set a time to think about the issue. Not necessarily a time— no need to whip out your daily planner—but give yourself permission to completely forget about the issue until then. When the problem has been delegated to a future time slot, you will be free to delve more deeply into the twists and turns of the sensual experience at hand.

Another possibility is spending more time unwinding before you get sexy—a hot bath, a little lounging around, a neck massage, or even taking a minute to appreciate your own innate sexiness is more than enough to break free of these thoughts.

All you can think about is an attractive person who is decidedly not *the one going down on you.*

Oral sex is particularly well suited to fantasizing. Because you can relax and can't see much of your partner from most positions, it may well be Tom Cruise or Salma Hayek (or for the really imaginative, both) giving you the ride of your life.

For most people other-person fantasizing is neither here nor there, but the fact that some people feel guilty about it is definitely here. If it bothers you, you may find that relaxing and focusing more deeply on your bodily sensations actually removes the *need* for fantasy of any kind.

One option is simply to realize that your mind is wandering and to call it back to an awareness of your own body. Focus your attention on what you feel—this will make the oral sex better regardless. How do the sheets (or the carpet, or the dining room table) feel against your back? Notice your own body: How does the air feel on your skin? Are your nipples hard or soft? Rub your fingers lightly over your chest, noting the feel of your own skin. Sometimes we have to use simple measures to reintroduce ourselves to our bodies as a source of pleasure. Now refocus on the sensations your partner is giving you. Propping yourself up into a sitting position and wrapping your hands around the head of your lover can be a great way to let your body tell your mind exactly where you want it focused.

If you're still feeling distracted, don't be afraid to stop your partner and tell them that you're having trouble relaxing. If you make it *your* problem, most partners will be happy to help you relax. A little massage or foot rub can sometimes be more than enough and may lead to some pretty exciting sex on its own. You may get an invitation to talk over your thoughts, which is usually just the thing to send them away.

But if you decide to tell your partner to stop, be mindful—phraseology is very important here. You may be saying "this sucks," but for the time being it needs to sound like "I'm distracted." For now, take responsibility for your response. Later, frame your criticisms ("you need to . . ." "you aren't . . .") as suggestions ("I think I might like . . ." or "I want to try . . .") Remember: the person giving oral sex is just as vulnerable as the one receiving it.

All you can think about is what bad thing you might smell/taste like.

As hang-ups go, this one is the most needless, if only because it underestimates your partner's freedom of choice. You wouldn't blame yourself if your lover decided to use some slightly turned milk in their coffee or wanted to eat a plate of something you personally found distasteful. What your lover puts in their mouth is a conscious and considered decision. Granted, if you have herpes (or any other STD) and this is the cause of your concern, then you should *definitely* speak up. Otherwise, unless you're getting it on with a first-timer, the likelihood is that your partner knows exactly what they're getting themselves into. And if they're going down on you, they clearly *want* to get into it.

In the event that this abstract "freedom of choice" talk doesn't do it for you, the other option is to simply tell your oral sex lover to "hold that thought" and go to the bathroom. If the courtesy of cleaning yourself will ease your mind, then it's well worth the interruption. Either way, if this is a concern of yours, make sure to do away with it before it does away with your good time.

All you can think about is the mound of cellulite/big pimple/strange and winding ass hair you discovered this morning after getting out of the shower.

Before a date, women and men alike will despair over one aspect or another of their physical appearance. And when clothes hit the floor, it's rare not to have a moment of exhilarated fear. Covering up our smells with deodorant, shaving off unsightly hair, clipping away our nails and painting our faces with little brushes may make us more palatable to ourselves, but the message it conveys is that the natural body is unsavory and even gross. And how can you feel excited about showing your lover something that must be continually repressed? Something that has to be regularly washed and wiped because it is constantly getting itself gross again? And the licking is going to be happening where?

Aside from all the reasons, cultural and personal, why we may be self-conscious about our bodies, the important thing to remember is that we are *all* self-conscious about our bodies. Bottom line: the intense self-consciousness that comes with the first few sex events renders most people as blind as a bat. So you might as well enjoy yourself, and try focusing your energy on your partner and your pleasure.

When it's worth the sweat, sex temporarily lobotomizes our capacity for abstract analytical or critical thinking. And yet most people fear being criticized, analyzed, and examined precisely during these sensual and engrossing experiences. Sometimes I think my partners wouldn't be able to tell me how many fingers I was holding up during sex (though the experiment has never seemed worth the interruption).

You're Afraid of What They Might Do

Remember that your partner only has one goal in mind: to give you pleasure. So let them succeed by really relaxing and enjoying yourself. If your partner is worth their salt, they will be trying to figure out your comfort zones by tentatively exploring areas and then waiting for cues from you to continue or not. Enjoy the preliminaries, and if you start to feel frozen up or like you're not responding, have them return to something you liked earlier. A little sigh or grunt will usually be more than enough to get your message across to a good partner. Others may have to be physically reminded of what felt good with a gentle nudge. The best partners will be on the lookout for shifts in your body posture, breathing, and muscle tension and will change their techniques accordingly.

Another option is to nip your discomfort in the bud by showing your partner what you like. You can use your hands, mouth, or anything else you can think of to demonstrate. You can also use hot, sexy language to describe it in a way that will build anticipation. A girlfriend of mind had a pillow that resembled a vagina, and she used to point to it to indicate what she liked. It had a lot of comedic appeal, but some people definitely need explicit instruction, so don't be surprised if one of them shows up in your bed.

You should never have to feel concerned or tense about what your partner might do to you during oral sex. A few words, and sometimes just a subtle movement, are enough to give them the indications they need for what makes you comfortable and what you like.

Now that you're truly prepared, inside and out, to give and receive oral sex (and perhaps do both simultaneously), let's suit you up with the skills you're going to need to capitalize on this potential for a deeply satisfying sensual exchange.

3

Initial Tonguework for
Lingual Love

PREPARING YOUR MOUTH AND TONGUE
TO MEET YOUR PARTNER OF CHOICE

BEFORE BEGINNING THE exercises, let's take a moment to isolate and define the problems you might be addressing with them.

1. *Lockjaw.* Your jaw is gripped by tension, set in one position, so your tongue is allowed no free play. (This can be a particular problem for lispers.)

2. *The Tooth Monster.* Lack of jaw control can mean that your teeth get in the way, snagging on things that they shouldn't and making what should be a tender, erotic moment seem like an operation without anesthetic.

3. *The Drowning Pool.* You produce too much saliva, which gets in the way of your breathing properly and keeping up a steady, even, controlled stroke.

4. *The Tongue Depressive*. Your tongue is sluggish, lazy. You can't flick it lightly to catch those sensitive spots at the right time and with the right pressure.

5. *Flabby Tongue*. Your tongue is bulbous, large and flaccid, with no flexibility and no tonal quality. For all the good it does your partner, it might as well have rolled itself up into a ball and curled away to hibernate for the winter.

6. *The Big Gag*. You don't know exactly why, but you're gagging. And you thought only collard greens could do this to you! But don't worry, it can be easily fixed without years of psychotherapy.

Everyone has a different relationship to oral sex, and while many of these problems may have psychological and cultural components, developing your skills and sense of confidence toward oral sex will help give you an overall sense of well-being. If some or all of the issues mentioned apply to you, you might want to jump ahead to chapter 6 and take the Oral Sex Fitness Test. Then, when you have a sense of how fit your tongue is in general, you will know how often to perform the exercises needed to strengthen the following areas and eliminate these problems for good.

The techniques you're working to attain will create a firm foundation from which you can build more advanced skills. They won't automatically make you a great oral lover, but they will give you all the tools you need.

Jaw Control. So you can open your mouth as wide as necessary, without straining.

Proper Breathing. Learning how to breathe in and out through your nose, so you don't run out of breath while your mouth is busy.

You'll eliminate one more distraction, and make it that much easier to concentrate on the magic that's passing between you and your lover.

Easing the Tension. Oral sex involves more than just your mouth. Learning how to relax your neck and shoulders, your knees, your fingers, your whole body, will contribute greatly to your being able to focus all your enthusiasm on the matter at hand.

Swallowing. Using your whole throat to swallow releases the constrictions in everything that's above it—tongue, sinuses, nasal passages.

Tonguemanship. This is probably the most sensitive, sensuous part of your body. But you have to know how to use it—and you have to get it into shape.

GETTING TO KNOW YOUR TERRIFIC TONGUE

The next time you're in the bathroom, take a look at your tongue. Most of us think of our tongues as one unit, but the tongue has four distinct sections that you will need to familiarize yourself with in order to move your tongue techniques into second gear. These are: the tip (the position of the tongue nearest the teeth), the blade (the point just below the alveolar ridge), the middle (the section that touches the roof of your mouth when you arch your tongue by placing the tip behind your lower teeth and pressing upward), and the back (the part that falls away from the roof of your mouth in an arched position).

Your tongue is the largest and most powerful muscle in the body and is distinguished from other muscles by its ability to flatten and point itself so dexterously. Because of its capacity to flatten and lengthen, or sharpen and point its tip, as well as its ability to alternate between heavy and light exertions of pressure, the tongue is custom-crafted to administer oral sex. There is nothing else in the sex shop that can do all this. To boot, the tongue has a smooth underside, as well as a rough top texture "for their pleasure."

The Spot

The first step in developing your tongue's strength and precision (directly connected to its ability to give pleasure) is to identify the Spot. This is a particular place on the roof of your mouth where you will need to place your tongue for the majority of the tongue- and lip-strengthening exercises in this book. To find it, insert your (clean) finger into your mouth so that you're touching the place where the backs of your top teeth meet the gums. Trace your finger from here to the spot where the roof suddenly drops to another level. This slope is known as the alveolar ridge.

Remove your finger and start playing with your tongue. See how sharply you can point the tip. It needs be more like a pencil than a hot dog. The sharper you can make the tip, the more delicately and precisely you are going to be able to stimulate your lover. (If you can't make a well-defined point now, don't worry; there are exercises later in the book that will help you develop one.) When you have made your best possible point and identified the tip of your tongue, place the tip *only* on the drop-off (or alveolar ridge). Don't let your tongue touch your front row of teeth, and make sure that it doesn't fall beyond the ridge.

Keeping your tongue in this position will stop it from changing the position of the lips, something the tongue is notorious (in my field anyway) for doing. Think of your tongue as a hammy actor—it's always trying to get past, distract, or upstage your lips and jaw from

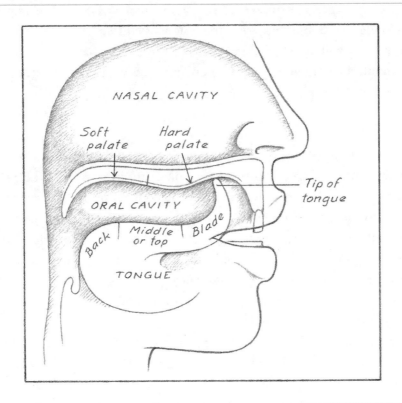

The Spot: Perfect Placement for the Tongue

their function. But worse than that, it can also take energy away from the lips. So put that tongue in its place.

Aside from enabling you to participate in the exercises, placing your tongue here can stimulate the blood supply to the brain, increasing concentration and mental clarity. To do this, keep the tip of the tongue pressing up into the Spot, and let the middle of your tongue come up onto the roof of your mouth *without* changing the tip's pressure. Only the middle should be pressing into the curved top of the mouth. The back of your tongue should still be hanging down into the back of the mouth. Holding this position will help you become more composed and clear-minded. It requires a little practice to keep your tongue here (about as much as teaching a dog to stay), but this position gives back ten times what you put into it.

4

Kissing

Graze my lips, and if those hills be dry,
Stray lower, where the pleasant fountains lie.
—WILLIAM SHAKESPEARE,
"Venus and Adonis"

PERHAPS BECAUSE KISSING on TV and in movies is immediately passionate, kissers tend to try to copy what they've seen. But the art of kissing cannot be reduced to pucker-and-lunge. There are as many different kinds of kisses as there are people kissing, and each has its own particular combination of pressure and pace.

The ancient Indian *Kama Sutra* was aware of this and devoted an entire chapter to kissing, identifying fourteen types of kisses. In our culture today, we seem to have forgotten just how varied kissing can be. We know about the peck, the lip kiss, and frenching, but everything in-between is frequently overlooked, and kissing itself is frequently rushed through as if it were a trifling preliminary.

This may be in part because most of us don't know how to use our mouths and lips in ways that produce a variety of erotic, pleasurable sensations. (Though erotic desperation definitely takes some of the blame.) Whatever the cause, maximizing the pleasure afforded by your kisses will enhance all your lingual caresses and alert your partner to the pleasures in store for her.

The most common complaints I hear concern half-lipped, lifeless kisses, so we'll address these first. Complaints about this kind of kiss range from disengagement ("I felt like she was just poking and pressing her lips around mine") to actual confusion ("It seemed like he was trying to whisper something really close to my mouth, like right into it . . . then I realized he was *kissing* me"). A very common phenomenon, this kind of weak kissing results from the individual using only a small portion of the outer lip to kiss, instead of their full lips (including the smooth insides of the lip). The result is a dry kiss that feels more like lip bumper cars than an expression of passionate tenderness. The exercises below will help you use your full lips to create a maximum sensation of pleasure when you kiss.

COMING TO GRIPS WITH YOUR LAZY LIPS

Though they take over completely during kissing, lips are a primary point of contact with your lover during all of oral sex and so must be as exquisitely soft and pleasing to the touch as possible. These kissing exercises must be as devoted to developing a velvet touch as they are to extending and strengthening lip movement. While developing mastery over the movement of the lips is extremely important to help them create a wide variety of sensations on cue, you never want to tone your lips so much that they become too firm or muscular.

To keep your lips soft and inviting, make sure that you *never* perform lip exercises with tense lips. Pucker and tap your lips gently with your index finger. How soft do your lips feel? This is how they should feel when you perform the lip exercises. Avoid tensing your lips when you go through the motions of each exercise. For the first week of practice, you should do all of the exercises standing in front of a mirror, so that you can be sure that the correct parts of the lips and mouth—and nothing else—are moving. In the beginning, you should do each exercise separately, with a five to ten minute break in between. After the first week, the exercises can flow into each other. Each exercise should be performed every day for seven days to start, then switch to every other day for an additional week to train the muscles to remember their new skills.

Kissing Exercises

Pucker Up

With your tongue on the Spot (see chapter 3) push your lips all the way forward until they open and roll their insides out, sticking as much of the inside of your lips out as possible. Then, keeping them fully extended, open and close your lips, bringing just the fleshy parts together to form a small circle. Touch them together five times.

Practicing Pucker Up may make you look a little silly, and a lot like a fish, but trust this exercise—it will put you far ahead of the game by helping you find the correct positioning of the tongue and jaw.

This exercise acquaints you with the soft insides of your lips—when you perform it, notice what potential the lips have to create soft, delightful sensations. Lip implants are popular because they promise exactly this sensation. But in order to deliver it, make sure to note the difference in texture between the soft, glossy inside and the drier outside of the lips. Many people make the mistake of firming up the lips, and kissing with only their rough outside edges, thereby missing out on the moist inner lips' inherent kissability. (You can feel how unstimulating this is if you simply close your lips and slightly roll them in between your teeth so that only the outer lip is exposed.) This part of the lip has no friction or engagement, both of which are absolute necessities for an erotically stimulating kiss.

However, others make the mistake of rolling the lips out too far. This results in the "I felt like he was eating my face" sensation. When you kiss, the other person should be able to feel *both* the rough and glossy parts of your lips and never just one or the other. Similarly, during oral sex, the entire lip should be used for greatest effect. However, on a particularly sensitive clit, use just the glossy insides to avoid over-stimulation.

Another issue that significantly impacts kissing and oral sex is the *strength* of the lips. Most of us never think of the lips as muscles, but lip strength is an extremely important factor for any kind of lingual caress. Pucker Up identifies and prepares you to use your entire lips, but if the muscles are weak the effect won't contribute much to your kiss. In order to give a really memorable, arousing smooch, your lips need to be strong and under your control. One exercise for this is called E like "Eat," O like "Swoon." (You can use your imagination for what kind of "eating" this refers to.)

E *like "Eat,"* O *like "Swoon"*

With your tongue on the Spot and your teeth together, look at yourself in the mirror and pull your lips as wide apart as they can possibly go. Place your pointer and middle finger with the pads against the teeth, and start saying "eeeeeeeeee." Not "ehhhhhh," like "elephant," but a strong, sharp "e" like "eat." Keep looking in the mirror to make sure that your lips are the only things moving (that is, don't move your jaw, neck, or tongue) and that they are stretched widely enough so that they aren't touching your fingers. Hold your lips in this position for the count of ten.

When you're ready, remove your fingers and pull your lips into a tight little circle with the insides of the lips pressing forward—as if you were trying to touch someone else with the smooth insides of the lips—and say "oooooo" like "swoon." This will strengthen your lips, as well as the surrounding muscles.

Do ten repetitions of these kissing exercises every day for a week. The more advanced exercises later in the book will build on them, both in chapters 7 and 10.

Once you've mastered the exercises specifically for kissing, you can start practicing those intended for the much more powerful king of kisses: oral sex.

Advanced Lip Exercises for Kissing

The Saltwater Pump—Front

Pumping exercises increase your lip dexterity. Put one teaspoon of salt in half a glass of warm (not hot) water. Pump a mouthful of this back and forth behind your upper lip. Allow the shape of your lip to be changed by the pressure of the water moving in and out. Perform this for a full minute, pushing the salt water as far as it will go without opening your lips. The presence of the salt will make you aware of the exact places your lip expands with this exercise. Take note of how much your lip can actually stretch, because you'll be using the insides of your lips extensively in kissing and manipulating the finer points of your lover's anatomy. You should be using a half a glass of water to complete this exercise through a series of three to seven mouthfuls (depending on the size of your mouth). Do this three times a day for a week.

Remember not to swallow the water. Stand nearby a sink or receptacle so that you can spit it out.

The Lip Massage

Whereas the Saltwater Pump softens the deeper tissues of your lips, performing the same motions with air softens the surface of the lips, especially the delicate edges where your lips touch. It will also help you gain control over this crucial area for oral sex. This is the part of the lip that will hold the clitoris in place; it is also the part of the lip that is most responsible for stimulating the surrounding area during clitoral stimulation.

Using your breath instead of water, push air behind your upper lip as firmly as you can. Again, do not tense or engage the lip muscles, but allow them to be moved and stretched by the power of your breath. Do this ten or twelve times during the day.

The Saltwater Pump—Side

Using the same ratio of salt to warm water as in Saltwater Pump—Front, push the water outward against the cheeks. Allow your cheek muscles to relax completely, then slowly push the water completely into them and maintain the position for a few seconds. Let the water blow back into the mouth gently, with still further relaxation of the cheek muscles. Alternate forcing the water in and out of the cheeks in this manner. Do this five times a day, filling and emptying twice each time.

Monkey Face

Slowly force salt water behind the upper lip, gradually building up pressure until the lip is completely rounded out. Make sure that the lip muscles are completely relaxed. Do this five times in a row, then perform the same process on the lower lip.

Try this again using air to reach the subtler musculature. The reason for doing both is that while using water makes the lips more flexible, air makes them tangibly softer. Taking some air into your mouth, force it gently into your upper lip, as if you are blowing up a balloon. Hold to the count of ten, five times in a row on the upper lip, then the bottom lip, and then both.

The Jug of Plenty

This exercise will give you some of the softest, most memorable lips on the planet. To perform it, you need an empty plastic half-gallon jug (or container of equal size and weight) and about four or five feet of string. Good cotton string is highly preferable to dental floss or thread.

Place the jug on the floor, and tie the cotton string through the handle so that you can lift the jug off the floor with the string. Put one end of the string in your mouth, and bend over so that you are looking directly down at the jug. Lift the jug off the floor by puckering your lips and using them to pull the string into your mouth. Do not bite the string or use your teeth. (And you may want to close the blinds!)

Some people start to suck as if they were eating a long piece of spaghetti. Instead, actively use the *inner* part of the lips to pull in the string, hold it to the roof of your mouth with your tongue, and then use your lips to pull in another segment. Lifting the jug six or eight inches off the floor will do. Your face should remain parallel to the floor. Lift and lower the jug ten times (each time should only take a few seconds).

Be very careful when taking the string into your mouth. Do not perform this exercise haphazardly or while rushing.

Button Up!

The purpose of this exercise is to get the muscles of your lips to strengthen by working against themselves. The idea here is to tone the lip muscles by forcing them to adapt to increased stress.

For this exercise, you will need a button between the size of a dime and a quarter, and a piece of string as long as your arm. Thread the string through the button, and tie the ends of the string together. Pull the button with one hand and the string with the other until the doubled string is stretched taut. Place the button in your mouth, and position it equally between your top and bottom lip (but not touching your teeth). Holding the button with your dominant hand (left for left-handed, etc.), hold the string so that it is perfectly straight and even. Begin to pull your dominant hand slowly away from your motionless head with steadily increasing force.

The button will attempt to escape your mouth by forcing your lips open—don't let it. Pull harder until you find the point where you lose the button. Try to remember how far away your dominant hand is when it pops free, so that you can set your goal for the next time just beyond that point. Do this five times a day for seven days, then three times a day for another seven.

These exercises all help make the lips supple and soft, while maximizing their tone and energy so that they never tire of giving your partner pleasure. The energy you put into your lips here will show up in tenfold when it's time to give some luscious licks and kisses.

Tongue-Tied

Let's refine your control and fine manipulation of the tongue. For french kissing, an excellent exercise is to look in the mirror and bring your tongue fully to a point. Would *you* want to kiss your tongue? It should be a healthy pink. If your tongue looks whitish, or even yellowish, make sure to use a tongue scraper after each brushing.

Stick out your tongue and bring it to a point without touching your teeth or lips. Hold it in this position and make a mental note of its size and shape. Now relax and widen the tongue as much as possible, still without touching your teeth or lips. The first time you perform this exercise in the mirror, you may be surprised by just how versatile your tongue really is—it can stretch from a point less than half an inch long to four times that size without touching the teeth or lips. The concept of your tongue as a free agent, moving independently of your teeth and lips is particularly important for oral love, even crucial. While kissing, allow the tongue to move independently, but avoid making it sharp or pointed (at least until kissing has become extremely passionate and aggressive). Remember that a soft, wide tongue is much more inviting than a darting poker, and that each minute change of your tongue shape will be felt intimately by your partner.

ORAL ETIQUETTE

Straight men need to be emasculated. I'm sorry. They all need to be slapped around. Women have been kept down for too long.

Every straight guy should have a man's
tongue in his mouth at least once.

—MADONNA

Allow me to say it for you: *What?* How could someone as sexually
open and liberated (at least ostensibly) as the superstar Madonna have
such bitter, resentful feelings about men and kissing? But more im-
portantly: Why should there be any relationship between kissing and
being "kept down"? The statement is clearly emotional, and relates
the way having a man's tongue in her mouth made Madonna feel. It
seems highly likely that somewhere along the line, a tongue went too
far and too fast, and what should have been a pleasurable experience
became distasteful, unpleasant, and (it sounds) even disrespectful.

Though Madonna's feelings as expressed here are extreme, I would
venture to say that the feeling of a tongue playing tonsil hockey in your
throat is not an altogether uncommon experience. Madonna may see
it as a patriarchal show of dominance, but her kissing partner(s) may
have just been unskilled and too nervous (after all, they were kissing
Madonna) to control the speed, force, and extension of their tongue.

This is the tragic downfall of the overzealous kisser. Inadvertently
making someone suck on your big tongue is definitely one way to put
the flame of passion right out. It does not, let me repeat *not*, necessarily increase your partner's passion to push your tongue further into
their mouth. You need to follow your partner's indications to figure
out when this is appropriate and desired—and when it isn't. A good
rule of thumb is to feel how much of their tongue they are putting in
your mouth, gently add one-fourth of an inch to that, and there's your
limit. As long as you are following these signals, your kissing will be
pleasurable and a delight to remember, increasing your sexual appeal
and the intimacy between you.

At this level of kissing it is also very important to be mindful of your breath. If you have eaten smelly food that day, it will be difficult to hide now. Remember that garlic, onions, coffee, cigarettes, and other bad-smelling consumables might make this type of kissing unpleasant for your partner. Making sure to brush, floss, and apply balm if your lips are dry and cracked are amenities your partner is sure to appreciate.

Kissing: Practice for the Big Day Out

Once you have practiced the exercises earlier in this chapter for a week, and your lips are stronger, more flexible, and fully engaged, come back to this section for kissing techniques. Though I wouldn't suggest trying everything in the *Kama Sutra* (there are some sections on biting and scratching your lover that seem better left alone), this ancient book offers a valuable perspective on kissing that I have attempted to incorporate here. The wide diversity of kisses it recognizes points to an important insight: each kind of kiss has a specific *meaning*, and transmits something particular and distinct to your lover. Adopting this attitude toward both kissing and oral sex will enable you to read your lover's signs and signals and to respond appropriately.

Lovers are constantly sending each other messages, with every breath, every movement, and each gesture. Becoming aware of how these messages are transmitted, learning to recognize them from your partner, and sending them more clearly, is the stuff of great sex. The several hundred thousand subconscious messages lovers send each other in bed (and out of bed, too!) lend sex between two individuals its distinctive character and determine whether sex is mind-blowing or humdrum. Being aware that each of your sexual gestures sends certain messages to your partner will help you tap into the silent sensual dialogue between your bodies.

Kissing with Your Whole Self

On some level, your partner will intuitively sense your state of mind when you kiss them. They will sense your desire—or your distraction. Some people are more sensitive (or more willing to delude themselves) than others, so there will naturally be discrepancies in your lover's reception. Considering that the majority of communication is nonverbal,* and that the acts of kissing and oral sex in particular consist of a high level of physical contact in one area, it's safe to assume that you'll have trouble hiding much of anything when you're going down.

To become a great kisser the most important skill you can acquire is that of focus. When your lips touch your lover's skin, on the lips or elsewhere, make sure you are fully mentally present and not just going through the motions. Do whatever it takes to focus in on the part of yourself that desires intimacy with this person. Focusing on that part will make it blossom and will lead your eager tongue to spots divine. There is no inspiration so great as true comfort.

The types of kisses discussed below (roughly inspired by the *Kama Sutra*) should help you distinguish among the different types of kisses and become aware of all the different messages a kiss can communicate. It is set up according to levels of intensity, from least to most intense, and while generally that is the best progression for sex, it does not need to be followed to a T; rather, the best guide for what to do and when to do it is the response of your partner. Let your kissing me-

---

* Albert Mehrabian, *Nonverbal Communication* (Chicago: Aldine-Atherton, 1972). Mehrabian is credited with finding that only about 7 percent of the emotional meaning of a message is communicated through explicit verbal channels. About 38 percent is communicated by paralanguage (which is basically vocal intonation). Fifty-five percent, the largest segment by far, comes through nonverbal communication, which includes such things as gesture, posture, facial expression, etc. During sex, that arena is sharply narrowed to the act of touching.

ander and explore, returning to what works, and abandoning what doesn't without stress.

The First Kiss

For the first kiss, you might want to try a soft, tender kiss where the lips merely touch each other for a moment, without much saliva or motion, but making sure to use a little bit of the smooth inside of the lip. Essentially, what this kiss says is: "I think I might be interested in kissing you. Care to join?" This kiss has little to do with the position of the lips, and it doesn't need any complicated hokeypokey. It transmits a simple message of interest.

If your partner responds just a little, or not at all, to this gentle kiss, you should bide your time before progressing to a more forceful kiss. Generally, the best sign that your partner is ready for an increase in intensity is their body movement. If she's moving her lips, and her hands are starting to reach for you or rub you, or her body moves closer to yours, the light doesn't get greener.

The "Relax, I'm a Great Person" Kiss

If you just made a tentative First Kiss and your partner isn't responding much, but isn't pushing you away or turning their face from you, they could be a bit apprehensive. This could be for a variety of reasons, personal or external. Do not rush or force this person—a few very light and nonthreatening kisses on the cheeks, forehead, and hair, may open them up like a flower. Gentle conversing, good eye contact, and light embraces are the best ways to make your partner feel comfortable. These light little kisses say, "It's okay with me that you don't want to go further than this right now. I enjoy just being with you."

If correctly done, this kind of "I like just being with you" kiss will increase your sexual connection with your partner in spades. If done with too much pressure, your partner will either feel overwhelmed or so exceptional that they will be calling you for the next millennium.

The Good Enough for Seconds Kiss

This kiss is a step beyond the First Kiss, and consists of an explorative, repetitive touching of the lips that says "Hello, here I am," then withdraws, but comes back again as if to say, "That's good enough for seconds." Picture someone tasting a new kind of ice cream cone for the first time—at first their lips touch the ice cream for a second, then they pull back, decide they like it, and go in for more. This kind of kiss can make your partner feel very special and desired. If your partner is responding well, by moving their own lips, that is the cue that they are ready for a more intense kind of kiss.

The Shower of Kisses

These are light little kisses showered all around the mouth, and can even extend to the cheeks. These kinds of kisses express how much you like your partner, as if you find their entire being, not just their lips, wonderful and kissable. Again, don't move forward unless your partner is responding to your kisses with movement.

The Relationship Changer

This is a somewhat firmer kiss that clearly indicates your desire for your partner. Until now, the First Kiss, the testing kisses, and the Shower of Kisses have indicated strong liking and affection. This firmer (not forceful) return to the mouth is about more than affection and liking. It says, "I want you." This is the kiss that breaks platonic bonds. It is not a hard kiss, but is unquestionably somewhat stronger than the earlier ones, and uses the entire lips, pulling one or both of their lips into yours for moments at a time.

A good way to develop this kiss at home is with a pitted plum. Choose a plum that is not too ripe or soft. Cut the plum in half and take out the pit. When you're ready, squeeze the half-plum so that it shapes itself like a slightly parted mouth, and bring it to your mouth. Move your tongue beneath the top ridge of the plum, and then the bottom. Try pulling first the top edge, and then the bottom into your mouth with your lips. Use the insides of your lips to pull the ridges in. This exercise will teach you how to use your entire lips to engage your partner's mouth. As you pull in each "lip" of the plum, see if you can rhythmically suck and massage it, varying the pressure and level of suction, instead of simply pulling on it.

The Hollywood Kiss
This is the first kiss where your partner will need to open their mouth. You can try to nudge it open lightly with your mouth, but this movement should be light and gentle, not sudden or forced. If your partner opens to accept your mouth readily, let the insides of your mouths become indistinguishable and surrender to one another.

The Tongue Exploration
This kiss is not to be confused with a poke or a prod. The tongue should not be overly pointed or aggressive. Instead, the introduction of the tongue should be the silky and soft presentation of the tongue on and around the lips. Think exploration, not excavation. Simply run your tongue along and around your partner's inner lips, gently sucking their lips, one at a time, into your own mouth.

Using your tongue indicates a greater degree of intimacy between you and your partner, so be sure that your partner is comfortable with the introduction of your tongue into their mouths. Do not push your tongue past their teeth at this point. If you ever feel your partner pull away from you (even slightly), go back to something less intense.

The "I Want a Piece of You" Kiss

Once you sense your partner is getting excited and responding to your movements, you can start making your kisses firmer and deeper. The firmer you kiss your lover, the more loudly you are telling her how much you want her. Your tongue is exploring her mouth beyond the teeth, perhaps interlocking with the taste-bud side of her tongue, and your hands are starting to hold on with more force. Compare it to exclaiming "I want you!" right to your partner's face. In the same way that you wouldn't yell this to someone on a first date, you don't just jump straight into this kiss. It's appropriate when it is adding fuel to the fire, and not being used to ignite one.

The Love Anvil

This is a harder kiss that you give once you are 100 percent sure that your lover is so hot for you they can barely stand it. More rapid responses to your kisses, accompanied by little cries or moans, indicate that your partner's passion is hot enough to fry an egg—and that's the *only* time when it's okay to apply the ten thousand pounds of pressure. Use your tongue to essentially copy the rhythm of intercourse by rubbing it more passionately and with increasing speed against the taste bud side of your partner's tongue. Until now, your tongue should have stayed fairly wide, but it's okay here to point the tip a bit because the kissing has become more passionate and aggressive.

The Erotic Nibble

Now that your partner is chomping at the bit, feel free to chomp a little right back. A love bite can add sensation and eroticism to a kiss, but must be performed very carefully. Exerting control over your jaw, give your lover a little nip on the lip. Your tongue should be in the Spot for this action, because otherwise you will bite too hard or too softly. Keeping your tongue in the Spot maintains good jaw control, so that your bite can be both tender and firm. The idea here is not to actually hurt them, but to heighten their sensation. Before you try this with someone else, try biting the skin on your own finger first, so that you can get a sense of the strength of your jaw and the sharpness of your teeth. The Erotic Nibble is a powerful gesture; it says "I want to consume you."

Progressing from light kisses to more intense ones—with plenty of space and time afforded for reversions, impulses, and experiments—is a good model for performing oral sex. In the same way that you would not jump right into a heavy, deeply probing kiss, oral sex requires a build-up period where your lover is given a little time to get used to the contact.

5

Oral Sex Ground Rules

YOU WILL ALWAYS have to customize oral sex for your partners: each person has a distinct set of preferences, and there's no getting around that. (We'll talk later about how to identify what those are.) But regardless of who your partner is, there are some base guidelines that lay the foundation for great oral sex.

LEND THAT HELPING HAND

There are two ground rules that need to be practiced constantly during oral sex. The first of these is that you should be using your hands, whenever they're not being used to prop yourself up, to caress and touch your partner. Oral sex centers on the tongue, but your hands and their ability to stimulate your lover by caressing, penetrating, massaging, and stroking should never be forgotten or overlooked. You won't hear me telling you to "move and caress with your hands" in the following pages, because it would have to be written on every single page.

EYE CONTACT IS CRUCIAL

The second basic ground rule is to keep reestablishing eye contact the entire time you perform oral sex. Make an effort to be constantly open, aware, and responsive to *all* of your lover's signs and signals. This is the best way to give truly satisfying oral sex.

DROP THAT 'TUDE, DUDE

The next ground rule has to do with attitude. In a Western, rationalist culture, it should come as no surprise that sex is often treated as a linear progress: "Partner wants orgasm. If I perform actions x, y, and z, they will result as quickly as possible in orgasm." But when has an itinerary ever made something more fun? The first step to giving truly memorable head is dropping the single-minded concern that your partner has an orgasm. Instead, try refocusing your energy on your partner having *fun*—at every stage of the process.

YOU MUST BE CLEAN FOR SEXUAL CUISINE

A few oral sex preliminaries. In addition to your general hygiene, pay particularly close attention to the following areas: Make sure that your lips are soft and supple to the touch, and apply cocoa butter or another moisturizer or lip balm to them if they feel rough. If you have facial hair of any kind, make absolutely sure you have a fresh shave before performing oral sex. If the hair has grown out long enough to be soft, fine, but a forty-eight-hour-old shave is downright inconsiderate. Finally, if you plan on using your hands extensively—as you are hereby encouraged to—either make sure that your nails are clipped close to your fingers or be hyperattentive to how and where they touch your partner's skin. And before you go down, brush those teeth. Brush 'em long and hard. Their bacteria can give her problems later.

RHYTHM NATION IS YOUR SALVATION

Another basic has to do with rhythm. Unless your partner is having a wild hormone surge, her genitalia will be easily overstimulated by sudden movements. Oral sex should always begin with light, gentle touches, kisses, and licks on and around the genitals to prepare the area for heavier stimulation.

GREEN MEANS GO, RED MEANS NO, AND NOTHING MEANS . . . ?

If your partner doesn't respond to the basic, introductory moves outlined above, never, ever simply proceed. You will feel uncertain, and this will affect your performance. The best thing to do in this situation is to pause and ask how she likes it (in a confident, inviting voice). If she says she doesn't know, ask her how she feels about trying some different things, or if there is something she would like to do instead. If she's open to it, this is a great opportunity for you to experiment with different light moves, and the orgasms of a doubtful partner will make you doubly proud. However, if she responds to your question with specific directives, treat it as a learning opportunity. She may put some signature moves in your pocket.

6

The Oral Sex Fitness Test

HE TEST GETS its own chapter because you will need to keep coming back to it to check your progress. These test questions will determine whether or not you are ready to proceed to the next set of exercises or if you need to keep practicing the exercises in chapters 3 and 4. All questions are yes or no; answer them as accurately as you can, then add up the number of yeses and read the explanation after the end of the test. This is not a difficult test—it may be the coolest test in history.

THE ORAL SEX FITNESS TEST

1. Can you make a well-defined point with your tongue? It should point straight out like an arrow, straight ahead, parallel to the ground. Try it standing in front of a mirror. Close your eyes, stick your tongue out, and try to point it. Now open your eyes and check its configuration.

2. Does your tongue rest in the Spot, as identified in chapter 3? Your tongue has *one* correct launching pad in your mouth.

Locate the Spot; then see if your tongue returns to it naturally.

3. Can you touch the corners of your mouth with the tip of your tongue—not the sides—on the first try?

4. Can you move your tongue independently of your jaw? Try this as a test: With your tongue down behind your lower teeth, pronounce a hard "k." Your jaw should open. With your tongue on the Spot and your finger lying lengthwise between your teeth with the tip pointed, pronounce the letters "n," "l," "t," and "d." The middle of your tongue should rub the roof of your mouth. While you're doing this, does your jaw move? Does your tongue touch your finger? They shouldn't. Stand in front of a mirror and say "cunning." If your jaw moves, you are not working your tongue independently.

5. Can you open your mouth, protrude your tongue slightly, then life your tongue into contact with your upper lip while keeping your mouth open?

6. Can you pronounce "t," "d," "l," or "n" without touching your teeth? Can you pronounce any of the above sounds, or "h" or "s," without your tongue protruding between your teeth?

7. Can you groove your tongue?

8. Do you sleep without snoring?

9. Can you whistle with your tongue without pursing your lips?

10. Can you put your finger to the back of your mouth without gagging?

11. Do you typically avoid sore throats and colds in the winter?

12. Can you press your upper lip against your nose?

13. When you pucker them are your upper and lower lips the same widths?

14. Do you breathe while chewing?

15. Do you chew your food well before swallowing?

16. Can you eat a bowl of dry cereal without milk? Can you eat comfortably without drinking?

17. Can you speak without lisping?

18. Can you speak in any situation without stuttering?

19. Do you speak clearly, without sounding nasal?

20. Can you keep your tongue on the roof of your mouth when you are not talking?

21. Do you have good-smelling breath?

These factors each affect your ability to give great oral sex. Count your yeses.

15–21: If you answered yes to more than fourteen questions, forge ahead! Your tongue has reached the level of agility it needs to perform the techniques and exercises in the next chapters.

8–14: If you answered yes to between eight and fourteen questions, you need to practice the exercises in chapter 4 for an additional nine to ten days.

0–7: If you answered yes to fewer than eight questions, stop in your tracks. You need to practice all of the exercises in chapter 4 until you can confidently answer yes to more questions. Return to this quiz as many times as needed to measure your progress.

7

Basic Mouth Exercises

No member needs so great a number
of muscles as the tongue; this exceeds all the rest
in the number of its movements.

—LEONARDO DA VINCI

THE EXERCISES YOU'LL encounter in this chapter each need to be performed a few times a day for one to two weeks. Essentially, once your musculature is built up, oral sex itself will maintain your progress. Until you've reached that merry mixture of practice and performance, you'll need to do the exercises about once a week to avoid regressing to old (and bad) mouth habits.

Are you annoyed when people ask you to touch your tongue to your nose—because you can't? Can you tie a cherry stem in your mouth? Are you incredibly turned on by those who can? Could you touch *only* the tip of your tongue to the corners of your lips, without touching the rest of your tongue to any part of your mouth? All of these moves are oral sex assets, and if you can't do them now, these exercises will help you on your way. Rolling your tongue is a genetically determined trait, so no amount of practice will help you there, but the others can—and will!—be cultivated. These movements of the tongue will be used heavily in advanced oral sex techniques, so take note. The tongue is a more complex muscle than you might think, and has a startling diversity of sensations to offer your lover. The following exercises will help you get in touch with all the possibilities.

But first things first: though you might not suspect that a tongue needs a warm-up, the techniques you will learn later will require a level of flexibility and suppleness that can only be achieved after some basic training. Skipping the basic exercises can result in tongue cramps and even lockjaw, so don't skimp on the prelims.

- Never, ever strain yourself while performing these or any other exercises.

- The entire warm-up routine should take between five and ten minutes.

- Perform the exercise once, except where indicated.

BASIC EXERCISES

Nose Touch
Stick out your tongue and curve it up. Try to touch your nose. If you can touch your nose already, try to touch only the tip of your nose using the tip of your tongue. Repeat twice.

Chin Touch

Stick out your tongue. Curve it down and try to touch your chin. See if you can touch your chin without the tip alone. Repeat twice.

Up and Down

Open your mouth, keeping your tongue inside and behind your teeth. Move it slowly up and down, touching the tip to the roof, then to the base. Do not run the tongue along the roof or over the teeth. Pretend there is a toothpick between the roof of your mouth and the bottom of your jaw, and move your tongue along this perfectly vertical line. See how fast you can go while keeping the tip as the point of contact.

Side to Side

Open your mouth a little. Let your tongue peek out. Move it back and forth to each corner of your mouth on a curved path (following, but not touching, your bottom lip). Do this four times.

Peanut Butter

Open your mouth a little. Pretend you have peanut butter all over your lips. Lick all the peanut butter off your top lip, then lick it off the bottom one.

Tongue Push

Keep your lips closed. Place your tongue against one cheek and push it out, while using three fingers to gently push against the tongue from the other side of the cheek. Repeat on the other side.

Open Wide

Open and close your mouth. Letting your tongue rest on the bottom of your mouth, stretch out your cheeks but don't strain your jaw.

Smiley Face
Keeping your lips closed, give the biggest smile you can muster. Think of the oral sex master you will shortly become.

Sad Mouth
Keeping your lips closed, turn your mouth down as far as you can. Think of the fact that according to the McKinsey Report 60 percent of women report that their spouses give "moderately" satisfactory oral sex.

Show Your Teeth
Keeping your teeth closed, open your lips and give a big smile. Say "extremely satisfactory" without touching your lips to your teeth.

Kisses
Pucker your lips and make one long kissing sound, keeping your lips closed, by sucking air in through your tightly contracted lips for ten seconds.

Raspberries
Stick out your tongue and close your lips around it. Then blow air out, letting your tongue and lips vibrate. This may tickle.

Pops
Press your lips together and pop them apart, making a loud noise. Do not suck in—the popping sound is created by simply rolling your closed lips in very slightly, then allowing them to separate.

Fish Face
Push your lips out to make a fish face (*without* sucking in your cheeks for dramatic effect). Open and close your lips a few times.

Lipstick Lady
Press your lips together and rub them back and forth, as if you are spreading lipstick around on them.

Oooooh . . . Aaaaah
Focusing all of your attention on your lips, very elaborately shape your lips into the small circle that accompanies an "oooooh" sound, and hold it for about ten seconds. Then, smoothly transition into opening your mouth as far as it will go and saying "aaaaah" for ten seconds. Do each five times.

If you have successfully completed these warm-ups, congratulations! They are admittedly hard for sophisticated adults to perform.

INTERMEDIATE EXERCISES

Now that your tongue, lips, and cheeks are soft, supple, and ready to move, you're equipped to practice more advanced exercises. These exercises apply directly to oral sex and simulate particular moves.

Tongue Cluck
Put your tongue tip behind your top teeth and get the sides of your tongue up, too. Suck in and cluck, making a horse-galloping noise. See if you can get the middle to come down first, and the tip of the tongue last.

Focusing on getting the middle of your tongue to come down before the tip will teach your tongue how to stimulate your lover using the soft underside of the tongue instead of the rougher taste bud side. Few people know how to do this, and as the smooth side of the tongue feels delightful on the sensitive parts of the body, this exercise is well worth the effort of mastering.

Tsk-tsk

Use this exercise to train your tongue to use the area between the roof of your mouth and the taste bud side of your tongue to create more surrounding sensations on your lover.

With your lips open, place your tongue tip on the bump behind your top teeth and suck in gently. If you hear a sound like a disapproving old woman, you're doing it right.

Whole Tongue Suck

This exercise helps you teach your mouth how to focus on a specific area and to use sucking to heighten sensation.

Suck your entire tongue up onto the roof of your mouth. Press and release, making a sucking sound. Repeat five times.

Tongue Stretch

This exercise will give your tongue more dexterity, so that you can be sure to find your lover's hot spots.

Place your tongue on the roof of your mouth while you raise and lower your jaw. You should feel your tongue stretch. Repeat ten times.

Tongue Push

With your lips open, push your tongue onto the bump behind your top row of teeth for ten seconds. Relax. Repeat three times.

This will teach you how to apply pressure with your tongue in a designated place, and it will strengthen your control over when and where your tongue applies force.

Baby Talk
Place your finger between your top and bottom rows of front teeth and practice saying these syllables: "tuh, tuh, tuh, tuh"; "duh, duh, duh, duh"; "nuh, nuh, nuh, nuh." Notice how your tongue moves

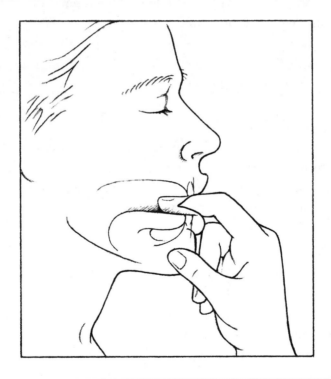

The Tongue Push

down with the center first, and then the tip? This will help you further develop your ability to stimulate your lover using the soft underside of the tongue. Your finger should have no teeth marks on it, and should not be wet by the end of the exercise.

Crush That Candy

Using a small piece of circular candy (like a Skittle or M&M), use your tongue to press the candy into the bump behind your front row of teeth, without pressing your tongue into your teeth as well. Press the candy with your tongue steadily, until it breaks or dissolves. Do not repeat. For the health conscious, a Cheerio works exceptionally well.

This exercise tones and strengthens the tongue, and if practiced regularly, will eliminate fatigue.

KKK (Not That One)

Keeping your tongue tip down behind your lower teeth, open your mouth and make a "k-k-k" sound by lifting the back of your tongue. When your lover is ready for more intense stimulation, use this tongue motion to stimulate them with the rough, taste bud side of your tongue.

More Imaginary Peanut Butter

Pretend you have peanut butter all over your bottom lip. Stretch your top lip over your bottom lip and pretend to wipe all the peanut butter off, addressing the sides as well as the front.

For supersensitive areas on your lover, the lip is a great substitute for the tongue. The soft inside of the upper lip can extend in the manner exercised to caress and awaken sensitive spots that can be stimulated more aggressively with the tongue later.

Hold It and Blow

Practice blowing a cotton ball across a table through a straw held firmly between your lips. Focus on applying specific amounts of pressure with the air you exert from your mouth. This will both fine-tune the muscles of your mouth and teach your tongue to flatten at just the tip—an excellent position from which to initiate upward strokes over the clitoris (or other supersensitive areas) with definite feeling but not an overwhelming degree of it.

Different Strokes

Pretend that you have whipped cream all over the roof of your mouth. Using the tip of your tongue, sweep it from front to back along the roof of your mouth. Do this for ten strokes, then change direction, now going from front to back and noting the difference in sensation.

The basic exercises should be performed for two weeks, and the intermediate ones for an additional week. (This is because the intermediate exercises build on and hone the raw skills developed by the basic ones.) Take the Oral Sex Fitness Test in chapter 6 to figure out whether or not you're ready to move on.

8

An Anatomy Class You Need to Pass

> The tremendous sea itself, when I could find
> sufficient pause to look at it . . . confounded
> me. . . . Undulating hills were changed to valleys,
> undulating valleys were lifted up to hills . . . every
> shape tumultuously rolled on, and beat another
> shape and place away. . . . I seemed to see a
> rending and upheaving of all nature.
> —CHARLES DICKENS,
> *David Copperfield*

UNFORTUNATELY, MANY PEOPLE feel confused when confronted with the structure of the vagina. It doesn't come with an instruction manual, and its parts and functions are far from self-evident. (After all, it's closed off and covered in hair—not as user-friendly as the plain-sight penis.) But in order to give a really good *mange*, her vagina has to become *your* vagina. In sexuality as in life, knowledge is power, so let's get down there. Do your best to memorize all these different parts, because you can't go whipping this book out between the sheets.

THE VERSATILE VAGINA:
THE MANY PARTS AND THEIR MANY PLEASURES

When it comes to female anatomy, the parts basically divide themselves into two camps: Easy to Find and Major Jaw-Aches. We're going to begin with the *clitoris*, because even though it can be difficult to locate, its primacy in oral sex demands a lengthy treatment (both in this book and in the bedroom). From there, we'll move through the parts and places that are easy to find (*labia majora*, *labia minora*, *mons pubis*, *anus*, *perineum*, and *vaginal canal*), and finish off with the ones that can be more challenging to locate (the *urethra* and the *G-spot*).

The Essential Clit

What is the clitoris? The small budlike being wears a hood, so it's no wonder if you've had a little trouble getting a positive ID. The top of the vagina where the lips come together is clit territory. In order to expose it, pull back the juncture of the two lips (using two fingers is easiest) to expose the little sucker. (Or in this case, the suckee.) When she's aroused, the bud expands, reddens, and emerges to draw your attention.

The clitoris is a primary source of erotic stimulation, and most women can have orgasms from clitoral stimulation alone. Biologically speaking, the clitoris is the equivalent of the penis, as for the first few months after conception, the genitalia of male and female fetuses seem to be identical. Obviously, many changes follow, but the clit shares certain traits with the penis: it is exceptionally sensitive and must be

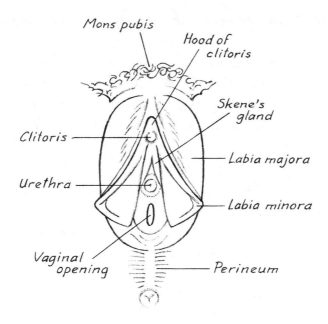

Mons pubis

Hood of clitoris

Skene's gland

Clitoris

Labia majora

Urethra

Labia minora

Vaginal opening

Perineum

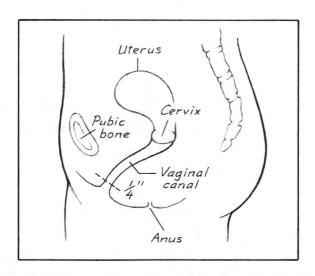

Uterus

Cervix

Pubic bone

Vaginal canal

$\frac{1}{4}''$

Anus

Female Anatomy

handled with care. When you touch the clit for the first time with anything but your tongue, lubricate whatever is coming into contact with it, from finger to vibrator (which, to avoid overstimulation, should not be turned up yet,) to whatever else you can think of. Just as continued stimulation after orgasm is painful for some men, rubbing the clit too suddenly or directly is anything but pleasurable. And do not bite or scratch it, ever. (If this needs to be explained to you, maybe you should stick to masturbation.)

Think Outside the Clit

While the hood may seem like a specialized clit-hider, it can work for you and with you as you stimulate your woman. And there's a good reason for its existence—a spot as intensely sensitive as the clit needs a shield from the world around it, otherwise women wouldn't be able to walk and talk at the same time. The best initial stimulation for the clit comes from *outside* the hood. Kissing, licking, and rhythmically massaging the hood will successfully stimulate the clit underneath and prepare the area for more direct stimulation. The clit is not a magic lamp to be rubbed until the orgasm genie appears. Instead, it must be approached gently, treated respectfully, and accessed in stages. Once it has been warmed up, it especially likes to be licked from the underside, though women differ in this regard. The combined activity of sucking and licking is the stuff of clitoral ecstasy.

How Do I Know the Clit Is Working with Me?

You can use your soft, lubed finger pads (with the nails cut or chewed away) to rub the clit gently, or your tongue to lightly lick it using upward, downward, or circular sucking strokes in either direction. Most women have a preference among these four methods, so trying each of them in the introductory phase and asking her which she prefers is a good idea. Many people think that if you don't know how to stim-ulate the clit, you should use your tongue to trace the letters of the al-phabet. As a last-minute default setting, this is fine, and may save you in situations where exhaustion or intoxication is a factor. However, af-ter you have read the following chapters, you will be a major *mangeur*. Once you've made the techniques herein your own, you will not need this "trick," except perhaps to buy some time while you decide which move is best suited to the occasion.

If you are stimulating the clit correctly, the vagina will get red, hot, and slippery, the clit itself will get harder and expand into something that feels like a pea, and your partner will be sighing or moaning. When one or all of these indications are in place (especially the vo-cals) feel free to give more aggressive strokes. Once she's approaching orgasm, make sure to maintain your rhythm and placement.

The Vaginal Canal

The entrance tunnel doesn't get much notice, but I single it out be-cause some women have extremely sensitive spots just inside the *vagi-nal canal*. These spots are located about one-quarter of an inch inside the opening, at eight and four o'clock. If you can explore these spots with your finger, that's great. If you can graze them with your tongue, that's even better. But be on the lookout for them.

Those Luscious Lips

Women actually have three pairs of lips, and only one of them is above the belt. The other two are both located in the vagina, and are called the *labia majora* and *labia minora* (fancy names for big lip and little lip). The labia majora is every bit as majestic as it sounds—these lips are the palace guards, protecting the *vulva* (another word for the entire vagina) from the intrusion of unwanted bacteria and objects. Partially because of the labia, the vagina is very safe from bacteria. Far from being dirty, it is actually cleaner than your mouth. Together with the labia minora, these lips work together to keep unwanted germs out, and to trap a great deal of your woman's natural lube *in*. In order to get a real reading on the state of all things lubricated, you have to get beyond the lips.

The lips extend from the pubic bone, or the *mons pubis*, to the *perineum*, the space between the genitalia and the anus. Remember these two spots, because they'll come out to play later. The labia majora can be pulled gently with the fingers to heighten early sensations, or sucked into the mouth with a gentle tugging motion. This indirectly gives a tantalizing wake-up call to the clit.

The labia minora is the inner lip that opens up in order for the vagina to be penetrated and that protects the especially delicate parts of the vagina—the urethra and the vaginal canal. These inner lips grow noticeably bigger and redder when aroused, and are more sensitive than the outer ones. They like to be stroked and massaged with a fair amount of pressure—unlike the clit, they can withstand a direct touch and even like it. While stimulating the clit with your finger or mouth, giving a good massage to the inner labia is a great way to heighten sensation and get the sweet sighs flowing.

If you can widen and flatten your tongue, the labia minor love to be licked in big strokes, with the soft, velvet touch available from the underside of your tongue, followed by a pointed explorative tip. (If you don't know how to employ this maneuver, practice the intermediate exercises beginning on page 60.) However, don't dwell on labia majora for two reasons: it is not as sensitive, and it is covered in pubic hair that you don't want to waste time spitting and picking out of your mouth.

If you have a penis—real or fake—use the soft rounded head to stimulate the labia minora by stroking these inner lips in long up-and-down strokes. If you have a vibrator, feel free to turn up the juice. Again, the labia minora is not as sensitive as the clitoris and likes to party. No tiptoeing around here.

The Urethra

I know, I know—it isn't a "sex organ," but the *urethra* is surrounded by highly sensitive nerve endings that play a part in your oral sex whether you're willing to admit it or not. When beginning oral sex, give a few quick licks in the space between the clitoris and the vagina to see if your woman is easily aroused by this sensation. If she is, study up. Medical literature contains plentiful accounts of women masturbating by inserting slender objects into the urethra, losing them during their bodily spasms, and having to have them removed by a doctor. We're not suggesting you follow suit, but it's an indicator that the urethra can be very sexy.

What Up, G?

What isn't, when the G-spot's successfully located? The *G-spot* is a treasure trove for the people who know how to find it. Its location depends on the woman, but hunting for it is a great use of time because the G-spot payoff never ends. Ever since this Grafenberg spot was discovered inside the front vaginal wall between the vaginal opening and the cervix, people have theorized that it is either a bunch of nerves related to the clitoris or a lube-producing gland of some sort. (I personally think of it as a reparations package for the period.)

Some women live and die by the G-spot orgasm, and very happily. Others prefer clitoral orgasms, and some prefer penetration, while others like a combo meal. It depends on your partner, and will take time and observation (or specific directives) for you to find out what she likes. (Men have a G-spot, too, located in a place that is best reached by vibrator or anal sex. See more on this in this book's companion volume, *Blow Him Away*.)

To start your G-experience, insert a couple of fingers into a warm, well-lubed vagina. Your palm should be facing up, so that the pads of your fingers can rub against the top of her vaginal wall. Gently and slowly bend your fingers forward (in a "come hither" motion) so that they stroke the front wall of her vagina. It may help to cup your hand so that your fingers curve without completely bending at the joints. You're not going to find something specific, but your girl might. Use your other hand to lightly press down on the outside of her stomach, so that you are adding pressure to the exploratory hand. You may find it useful to place several pillows under her hips or place her buttocks on your folded knees.

Remember, she might start howling with pleasure and ask you for a daily repeat performance, or she might just stare at you. There is no G-guarantee. However, using varying degrees of pressure and stroking styles will get you to the end of the G-spot rainbow—whether or not a pot of gold is waiting there.

If you have a G-spot vibrator, you'll notice that it's shorter than most and angles upward. Many people wind up poking these things in every way but the working one. The G-spot vibrator should never just be poked in. Hold it so that the curve is pointing upward with your hand grasping from underneath. Gently slide the tip of the vibrator in, and use a scooping-upward motion to move it in just a few more inches. Insert it slowly, using small circles or up-and-down strokes. When your woman goes off like a metal detector, make a mental note of your geography. You've just crossed the G-spot.

During penetration, the G-spot can best be stimulated by finding those positions which angle the dildo, vibrator, or penis so that it

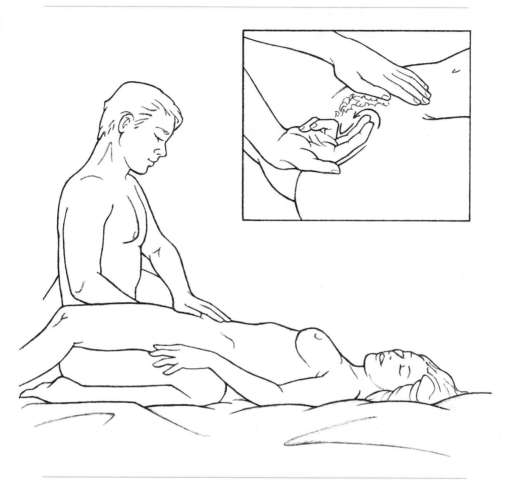

Find Her G-spot

touches the lower part of the front vaginal wall. A vibrator, dildo, or G-spot vibrator is ideal, because maneuverability is high and you can stimulate her clit with your mouth to heighten her G-spot glee.

For the penis, the positions that best access the G-spot will depend on its length, shape, and width. For a penis that curves up, the mis-

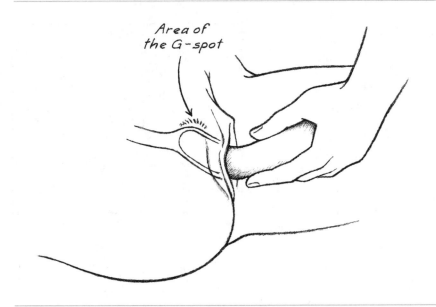

Area of the G-spot

Using a G-spot Vibrator

sionary position may work with varying levels of penetration. For a not-fully-erect penis, or one that tends to point straight out even when fully erect, rear entry or having the woman on top and bent very close to the man will work. If you're both in shape, you can also put the woman's legs over your shoulders. The key is having the G-spot itself higher than her other body parts. However, you can't give simultaneous oral sex from any of these positions. (If you can, that's one lucky girl you've got.)

No matter which area of her anatomy you are stimulating most successfully, remember that there are as many different kinds of orgasms as there are women, so don't go trying to use the same recipe on all your partners. Each woman has her own set of preferences, and it's up to you to communicate with her—both physically and verbally—in a way that is receptive to learning her likes and dislikes. You may have been with a clitoris-crazy woman or a G-spot junkie, but some women have vaginal orgasms, all-over body orgasms, and some even orgasm from thinking about sex too hard. So don't become too fixated on any one part of her anatomy—they all have their particular charms to be elicited and enjoyed.

Do I Look Like a Urinal to You? A Note on Female Ejaculate

Don't worry: it isn't really pee. Female ejaculate is a real and present phenomenon, but it isn't a danger, and it has nothing to do with urine. Scientists suggest that it consists of a substance most similar to semen. Some people find female ejaculate surprising or off-putting, but if women have been orgasming anywhere near you (and we hope they have), you've probably been baptized several times without even knowing it. Female ejaculate is harmless, nearly odorless, and should be considered a reflection of the intensity of your lover's pleasure.

Female ejaculate probably emerges from the Skene's glands, a special type of tissue that surrounds the urethra. This type of gland is notably similar to the prostate in men, which is perhaps why its product so closely resembles male ejaculate. Because it originates from near the urethra, many women hold back their ejaculate because the sensation resembles the need to urinate. Other women might stop it because ignorant partners have wrongly accused them of urinating in the past. It would be a shame to try to stop it because the fluid is followed by an orgasm considered by some to be more powerful than a man's. (However, I have always doubted that orgasms have a reliable system of measurement, and until a specialized seismograph is devised, those doubts will hold.) Suffice it to say that an orgasm accompanied by female ejaculate is something to celebrate.

The greatest known female ejaculate evoker is the G-spot. Stroking and rubbing the G-spot, while applying pressure with your hand on the lower abdomen to increase stimulation, will be sure to elicit the kind of orgasm that brings along female ejaculate. Keep in mind that not all women produce female ejaculate, and even the ones who do may not do so every time, while others produce a deluge that would make Moses back up.

9

Quitters Never Climax:
Breathing for Oral Sex

AND YOU THOUGHT it was just "through the nose." If you've ever run out of breath, or suddenly needed to stop during oral sex, this chapter is especially for you. Instead of gagging, running out of energy, or feeling like you've been on a three-day expedition to Mt. Orgasm, you can learn to breathe and control the muscles of your lips and mouth in a way that will keep you happy, comfortable, and energized for truly boundless oral sex.

Just because you can breathe well enough to keep yourself alive doesn't mean you're doing it correctly. Imagine someone hopping into a race car and joining a competition just because they have a standard-issue driver's license. Well, our bodies are equally complex and powerful, and it takes skill and know-how to handle them for peak performance. And unfortunately, most of us are treating our bodies like rent-a-wrecks.

PUT A TIGER IN YOUR TANK

Breathing properly is the fastest and most efficient source of energy available to a human being. Putting oxygen in your lungs keeps you alert, vigorous, and ready for physical activity. Unfortunately, it isn't as easy as it seems to pull air directly into your lungs. The only way to really get the air to come swiftly and directly into your lungs—rather than your stomach—is to breathe in through your nose with your lips closed, and that's not a habit most of us have truly acquired. Think about it this way: If you put food in your mouth, it goes into your stomach. Well, the same goes for air. Trying to breathe by putting air in your mouth is about as effective as trying to eat by putting food up your nose. Sure, a little bit will make it down there, but you need more than a little, especially when you're hard at work giving a good *mange.*

Vis-à-vis oral sex, there are several reasons why you should learn to breathe correctly. In order to perform oral sex for any significant period of time, you need to be able to pull lots of fresh oxygen in your lungs quickly and easily, without gasping or gulping. Have you ever been performing oral sex on someone and felt kind of like you were doing a bunch of work for nothing? You may give all sorts of interpretations to thoughts like these, but they're simple and natural responses to an insufficient oxygen supply to your muscles. Proper breathing can keep that oxygen flowing into the active muscles, which will keep you feeling good about giving your partner pleasure with plenty of extra energy to go on a riff when you get inspired.

I've included a quick and dirty regime to help you gain control and mastery over your breathing. It's basically divided into two parts, with two objectives. The first segment is made up of exercises to help you relax the throat and jaw muscles (making your lips, tongue, and neck more flexible and less likely to cramp), and the second section will help you make that relaxation involuntary through better breathing habits. Both sections will help your stamina and overall performance in the bedroom.

THROAT AND JAW RELAXING EXERCISES

Tension in the throat and jaw area is one of the most restricting factors to pleasurable oral sex performance. If your throat and jaw muscles are too tight, your flexibility and comfort will be compromised. These exercises will also help you develop a pleasant, powerful speaking voice.

If you have never practiced exercises like these before, you should do the Head Rolls first, before moving on to this. These exercises may seem simple, but they can have a very great effect on the state of these muscle groups, and so need to be practiced with care and caution. It is very easy to throw these muscle groups out of balance—I should know, because I've spent my whole life correcting them. So proceed gently, and don't start practicing *any* exercise too suddenly or vigorously. Remember: going slow and gently during the exercises will help you be vigorous and energized in bed, but doing the exercises slapdash and at breakneck speed will only hurt your performance.

Head Rolls

To relax the throat and jaw muscles, sit in a chair or on the floor with your back straight. Make sure the surface is hard enough to support a straight back, no matter what posture your head might be in. A good way to test this is to find a spot you think you'd like, then move your head in a circle. Does your spine collapse forward? This spot is not a firm enough surface. You need to choose a spot where you can move your head in a circle without significant movement in your spine.

When you've found a spot, relax your shoulders and let your head begin to roll to the right across your chest *without* exerting any energy. It's as if your head were a big balloon filled with water, and you are simply letting it roll forward. Exhale while your head rolls across your chest, then inhale as it starts to roll across your back. Feel the tension draining out of your neck and jaw. *Don't* try to stretch or strain yourself. No pressing, and no pulling. If you feel strain anywhere, restrict your motion to a smaller circle. Now reverse the direction, rolling your head to the left. Keep alternating direction every two or three revolutions, exhaling and letting your mouth open as your head leans back, inhaling and letting your mouth close as it comes forward.

Once you've started to relax the muscles of your neck and throat (about one minute) allow your tongue to swell and grow heavy in your mouth as you're rolling. You can even stick it out a little and let it come between your teeth. Allow your tongue to be so big and heavy that it can roll in the direction of your head. Practice for two or three minutes, three times a day.

This throat and jaw relaxing exercise is great because of its versatility—you can take a moment to practice it while sitting at your desk, waiting in the doctor's office, or even at a red light. The more you do it, the happier your throat and jaw muscles will be, and the less likely they will be to give up on you or wear out during oral sex.

TENSING AND RELAXING

This is a more systematic way to relax your neck, throat, and jaw muscles.

In a spot where your spine is fully supported and bending your head forward does not cause your spine to bend forward too, sit with your spine as straight as possible. The idea behind this exercise is very simple and very powerful: creating tension within certain muscles, and then releasing that tension. Most people are constantly storing their stress in the muscle groups of their neck and jaw area. When you consciously put tension into these muscles and then relax them, it gathers up all the other tension you stored in these muscles during your day and flushes it out, too.

For the next few minutes, you will be taking deep breaths in through your nose with your lips closed and tensing up a particular group of muscles for a certain amount of time. Then, with your tongue tip down and your mouth relaxed and open, you will exhale and release all the tension in those muscles while the air is flowing out. The most important elements are taking a deep enough breath—inhale slowly and fill your entire lungs—and knowing exactly which muscle groups to tense. This will entirely fill your lungs with fresh air—a rare treat for them.

Releasing Closed-Mouth Tension

With your tongue on the Spot (see page 30), take a deep breath through your nose, hold it, and close your mouth tightly at the same time. Press your lips together tightly, press your molars together tightly, and press your tongue into the Spot like there's no tomorrow. Increase the tension slowly but surely, until the muscles are as hard as rocks and as tense as they can possibly become. Hold for a count of ten, pressing with an extra push for the last count. Now, let it go! As the air flows out of your lungs, let all of the tension drain out of your lips, jaw, and mouth. Take a few breaths, concentrating on how relaxed those muscles are now that the tension has been drained from them. Give your head a little shake, allowing your face to shake like a rag doll, to release any leftover tension. Repeat, making sure to *let the air and the tension flow out of your mouth at the same time.*

Releasing Open-Mouth Tension

Be very careful with this exercise—do not do it if you have any pain in your jaw. With your tongue on the Spot, take a deep breath through your nose and open your mouth fairly widely until you feel the tension in your jaw hinge. Depending on the shape of your mouth, your tongue may want to come off the Spot, which is fine. At the same time as you're opening your mouth, stretch your lips forward as far as they will go. Increase the tension slowly, but don't open so wide that you feel any kind of pain. Hold for a count of five, giving a little extra push at the last count, and let go of the air in your lungs and the tension in your face at the same time. Close your mouth as the stress flows away with the air. Repeat, again opening your mouth fairly widely, and stretching your lips out as far as they will go. You may look a little like Mr. Ed getting ready for his feed, but the overall effect on your jaw muscles is tremendous. Yawning is a natural response to this posture— just let it happen, shake it out, and start over.

Take a couple of breaths before you go on, enjoying the sensation of relaxed muscles in your neck and jaw. This time, with your tongue on the Spot, inhale through your nose and start to stretch out your lips again. But this time, point your chin straight up. Feel a gentle stretching or a pulling being generated along your throat from the tip of your chin to about halfway down the length of your throat. Again, increase the stretch slowly without going to the point of pain. Hold your breath and stretch it out for a count of five, and then exhale and bring your chin back to neutral, letting the tension in your throat and lips flow out at the same time.

This time, you're going to put your tongue in the Spot, inhale, and lean your head forward and down to your chest. Press your chin firmly against your chest and feel the tension building in the front of your throat as you hold the air in your lungs. Build the pressure slowly, and again, back off before you reach the point of pain. Keep your chin pressed down, the air in your lungs, and stretch for a count of five. Let the tension spill out with the exhale. Repeat.

Releasing Upper-Body Tension
With your tongue on the Spot, inhale through your nose. At the same time close your eyes tightly, press your lips together, and bring your elbows tightly into your ribs, and hold your throat in a swallowing position. Inhale, lips closed, eyes closed, elbows pulled in, and—swallow! Hold for a count of three and let it go. Let the air out slowly, and the tension in those muscles should exit slowly with the exhaled air. Breathe in and out for a moment, just feeling the new absence of tension in those muscles. Repeat. Feel the relaxation in all those muscles.

Close your eyes and scan your head, neck, and upper body for areas where you personally might be storing excess tension. Do you remember a massage or physical therapist mentioning that there's a certain place where you tend to store tension? Those areas would be a great place to start. You should now take a moment to isolate those muscles and release their tension. Perhaps you tend to store tension in your shoulders—you can lift them up or pull them back and then release. Or maybe it's your stomach, in which case you can push out on the abdominal wall and then release. Choose whatever muscle group you feel could use a little relaxing.

Once you've identified an area where you're storing tension, inhale with your tongue on the Spot, hold your breath, and tense those muscles as tight as they will go without causing you pain. Hold and press for a count of three, then allow the air to leave your lungs, and let it carry out the tension with it. Repeat. Feeling and enjoying the release that takes place after each exercise is just as important as performing the exercises themselves, so take a moment after each one to appreciate the absence of tension in whatever muscle group you've worked on. These are two-part exercises, with pushing, stretching, and tensing forming one part, and relaxing, letting go, and releasing forming the other. You have to do equal amounts of each to maintain harmony and restore balance to your upper body.

Remember:

- Be careful whenever you exert tension into a push or a stretch. Build the pressure slowly, and never take it to the point of pain.

- Do these exercises with the written description to guide you for the first couple of days, but after that, feel free to practice them in the office, in the shower, or even on the subway.

- You will need to do these exercises two or three times a day for several days before you're ready to move on to the more advanced exercises in chapter 10.

For the first two or three days, just concentrate on how different all of these muscles groups feel while you exercise them. You probably didn't know how many different sensations and stress pockets you had in your throat and jaw. This is your equipment for making oral sex a true pleasure to give, so get used to it and treat it with care.

DEVELOPING A RELAXATION REFLEX

Now that you've gone through and systematically tensed and released the muscles in your neck, throat, and jaw for several days, you should be getting more and more conscious of the presence or absence of tension in these muscle groups. You should also be creating an association in your mind—and in your body—between the release of a deep breath and the release of physical stress. If that association becomes strong enough, you should become increasingly able to consciously trigger a relaxation reflex in the muscle groups you have worked with. This will prove to be incredibly helpful during oral sex.

If you regularly perform these breathing exercises, you will never have lockjaw or painful lips and muscles during oral sex again.

Let's do a little test to see if that reflex has already been established in your mind and body. Sit with your back straight and let your mind go back to the time when you were performing the tense and release exercises. Visualize yourself taking a deep breath, tensing your muscle groups, holding, and finally letting those muscle groups release their tension with the air in your lungs. Now prepare yourself to take a deep breath *without* tensing up any of your muscles. This time, when you have taken a deep breath with your tongue on the Spot and are holding the air in your lungs, use the time to allow your mind to simply scan your body for any tension. Concentrate on this tension so that when you exhale, you can let it spill out with the air. Feel the relaxation this inspires and repeat four more times.

Now you've established relaxation reflex that can help you anytime you're feeling stressed or tense. Muscle tension in the body makes oral sex uncomfortable and even painful to perform—neck aches, lockjaw, and buzzing or burning lips are all cured by performing these exercises.

Now that you've reached this point, don't leave the Head Rolls and Tensing and Relaxing exercises in the dust. Keep doing these exercises at least twice a day—they are positively wonderful for your mind and upper body, as well as for your respiratory system. But, in addition, two or three times during the day practice your relaxation reflex. This will be marvelous for your overall health and stamina. Whether you're walking into a high-pressure meeting or sitting down to dine on a first date, the relaxation reflex will help you be your calmest, most centered, and charming self.

Remember:

· When you're practicing the relaxation reflex, try to feel every ounce of tension flowing out of your upper body.

· It's extremely important to relax these muscles before performing the kind of strenuous oral sex that this guide will inspire you to.

· Always, always, always breathe in through your nose during these exercises, and keep your tongue on the Spot during the inhalations. If the tongue is down, it will block the air passageway and prevent the lungs from filling completely with air.

Though at first glance breathing may seem unrelated to oral sex, poor breathing is actually what makes oral sex uncomfortable for most people. When you're breathing correctly, you can soften and energize your face, neck, and lips muscles to an extent otherwise impossible to give limitless pleasure to your lover.

10

Serious Sexercises

THE REALLY CRUCIAL tongue exercises may be fewer in number, but they are the most potent exercises in the book. So if you're short on time and patience, this is where you should focus your attention. While most of the exercises until now have been fairly specialized, focusing on certain moves, techniques, and parts of the tongue and lips, these exercises are the quick 'n' dirty guide to getting maximum strength and flexibility out of your tongue.

Woman's Delight
This exercise is designed to train your tongue to rest in the most energizing position possible. The correct positioning of the tongue will also help you get maximum flexibility and range in the lips.

Place a Cheerio on the bump behind your top row of teeth, keeping it in place by pressing with your tongue. Now swallow, *without* moving the Cheerio. You will need to significantly increase the pressure of your tongue to stop the Cheerio from moving, thus building the strength and correcting the orientation of your tongue.

This exercise is so fundamental to developing an agile, capable tongue that ideally you should go through a whole bowl of Cheerios. Barring that, try ten to fifteen. (You'll know you're done with each Cheerio when it becomes soggy.) Try to keep your tongue in the same position for increasing periods of time—ideally, your tongue should always be in this position, lips closed, breathing through your nose.

If you have trouble breathing through your nose and often forget to keep your lips closed, try resting a twist tie between your lips. This gives your lips a "reason" to close, and you'll be alerted that your lips are open if it falls out. This trick will help you become more aware of your lips and their relationship to your breathing.

To supplement Woman's Delight, after you have practiced a few times, try to swallow keeping your tongue in that exact spot *every* time you swallow—regardless of what drink fills your glass or food fills your plate. These swallows are like push-ups for your tongue and are healthy for your whole mouth. The next time you go to give oral sex, you will be just as delighted as your partner is to see how masterfully you can create specific sensations.

Woman's Double Delight
This is essentially like Woman's Delight, except this time, you are going to use two Cheerios—one placed on the bump behind your top row of teeth, and the other placed about a half-inch behind that. The goal of this exercise is to activate the midsection of your tongue by getting it to keep the second Cheerio in place while you swallow. Don't swallow the Cheerios—the object is to keep them precisely in place.

After some practice, try to swallow this way every time. It will help your digestion as much as your oral sex skills.

Yet Another Delight
That's right—one more Cheerio almost in the back of your throat. Just do the three-Cheerio swallow a couple of times—if it's too difficult, that means you need to practice the previous two Delights. If it's easy, read up on the techniques discussed later in the book and go find your lucky lady.

Open and Close
Open your mouth as wide as possible and stick out your tongue as far as it will go. Make your tongue long and pointed at the tip, then draw it in slightly to shorten and widen it as wide as it will go. Repeat this five times.

Your tongue should be making two definite configurations: pointed and unpointed, wide and flat.

Oral Play
This exercise will give dexterity to your tongue and enable you to form and accurately employ a well-defined point.

Hold your lower jaw down with thumb and forefinger. Touch the tip of your tongue to the upper right molar, then the upper left molar, lower left molar, lower right molar, in that order. Raise your tongue to the Spot (see page 30). Lower the tip of your tongue to the roots of your lower front teeth. Repeat six times.

Open Your Jaw
Curl up your tongue and place it as far back on the roof of your mouth as possible. With your tongue locked in that position, open and close your mouth. Repeat fifteen times. This exercise will reteach you how to have control over the movement of your jaws and eliminate

involuntary movement, which creates the painful bites and sudden slackening of the mouth's movement that lovers tend to remember.

Getting in the Groove

Stick out your tongue. Now groove it. Bring it back into your mouth. Use a straw to roll the sides of your tongue on if you're having trouble. Repeat ten times.

Rolling Around

Place the tip of your tongue down behind your lower front teeth with your mouth open. Make sure it is touching right at the roots. Hum so

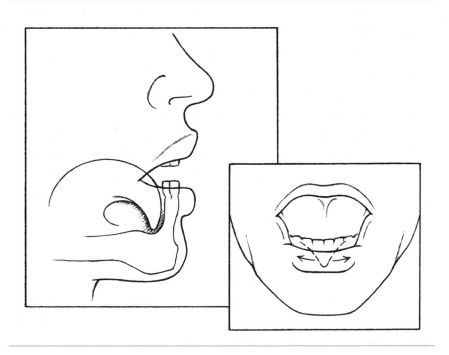

Rolling Around

the center of your tongue touches the palate. With the tongue in this position, rotate it from right to left. Watch yourself in the mirror to make sure your jaw doesn't move; this is a tongue exercise, not a mouth exercise. If your jaw moves, your tongue won't. This exercise will straighten and firm the muscles in the center of the tongue. Repeat five times.

Weight Lifting
Place the handle of a spoon on the center of your tongue. Keeping the spoon steady, push upward with the tongue and hold for a count of three. Relax the tongue between sets and repeat four times, three times a day. As you become proficient in this exercise, try to keep the tongue back in the mouth, perhaps just over the front teeth. This is the kind of weight lifting a girlfriend dreams of.

If you've completed these exercises, your tongue is the most agile, strong, and sensitive it's ever been, capable of quickly transitioning between feathery love tickles and intense, aggressive stroking before she has time to say "aah." But now that you have such a big strong tongue, what *are* you going to do with it?

11

Essential Oral Sex Techniques

ET'S SEE IF your brain is ready to catch up with your tongue. Remember the basic anatomy of the vagina? The clitoris, the G-spot, and the labia twins? What about the urethra and the vaginal canal? Perineum? Mons pubis? If not, try rereading chapter 8, An Anatomy Class You Need to Pass. These techniques will be much easier to memorize once you have the basic geography up your sleeve.

ORAL SEX 101

Remember that the secret to oral sex is sign language. Techniques are important, but knowing when and where to use them is doubly so.

Ladies First
If a man and woman are going to participate in oral sex, the idea that the man should perform on the woman first is not some residual act of chivalry. It is purely pragmatic. Women are capable of enjoying the

sex act and multiple orgasms for lengthy periods of time. A man typically takes time to rejuvenate after one single orgasm, and sadly, even
when rejuvenated, it can be difficult to muster the verve of the first
go-round. For this reason, the overall quality of oral sex goes up when
the woman can experience multiple orgasms through oral sex first,
and then the man can climb his own summit to exhaustion.

Dental Dams

A dental dam is essentially a small piece of latex (but you can use plastic wrap), which acts as a barrier between the vagina and the mouth.
Oral sex can transmit STDs, though there is less likelihood than with
intercourse. Aside from this general purpose, dental dams can be wonderful for people who are excited about trying anal stimulation, but
unwilling to "go there" without some form of protection. You can
really boost your oral sex technique by using a dental dam over your
woman's anus, and using anal stimulation to heighten her oral sex experience. But before we get into that technique, let's cover exactly
how you use them.

To use a dam, check to make sure that it is free of holes by holding
it up to a light or making sure that water cannot pass through it.
Lightly rinse the dam off with warm water and dry it with a towel.

Apply a water-based lubricant on your female partner. (This can be
a fun process in and of itself.) Only one side of the dental dam should
come into contact with the skin, so place the lubricant on the side of
the dam that will touch your partner. Cover the labia, vaginal opening, and clitoris with the dam, holding its edges with your hands, and
poke some of the dental dam into the vaginal canal. Then do everything exactly as you would have if she weren't protected. Use the
same procedure for protecting the anus.

Throw the dam away after each use, and never, ever switch a dam from the vagina to the anus or vice versa. You'd be putting your partner at risk for infection.

The feeling of a dental dam is distinct from that of skin, however the sensation is still very pleasurable. Usually, the person performing oral sex holds the dam so that their partner can lay back and enjoy the spreading sensations. There are those who believe that the partner should hold it, so that the oral sex giver can have their hands free for additional stimulation. Since this is a nonpartisan guide, I'll leave that choice up to you. There are also some dams that come with an adhesive strip to hold itself in place.

THE ESSENTIAL ORAL SEX EXPERIENCE

When you're ready to go down, make sure you take your fingers or sex toys out of the vagina for a few minutes if you've been fooling around. Take a moment for kisses and deep-dish necking like you just got home from WWII and give the nether regions some time to resensitize. (And on your way down, skip the whole blanket-over-your-head move. This seems sexy in movies, but will just make you overheat.)

A great way to heighten sensation before oral sex is to lightly and slowly run your fingers up the thigh area, then give gentle kisses around (but not quite touching) the genitals, perhaps running your fingers through or lightly pulling on the pubic hair. Before you dig in, switch to the other leg and perform the same inward trajectory, activating the nerves all around the genital area until you are lightly kissing and caressing the genitals themselves. This circling of the prey builds expectation and excitement. Once you begin caressing and kissing the genitals, remember that harder is not always better, and while

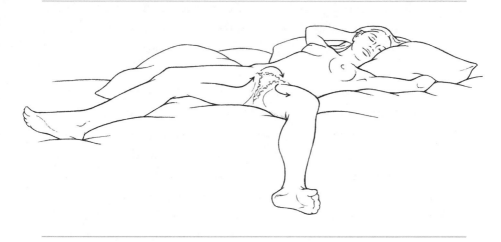

Stimulate Your Partner Before Diving In

a little saliva is an absolute prerequisite, sometimes less is more. (Too much saliva can actually dull sensation.)

When your partner begins to respond to these light touches—which can include blowing, licking, kissing, caressing, and even a little tickling—that is the green light for more speed and intensity. These are not *necessarily* most effective when delivered immediately. Being on the lookout for your partner's signs and signals doesn't mean you should be a sexual sycophant. Part of making oral sex more fun and less linear is the use of teasing, provocation, withholding, and whatever else you can think of to drive your partner nuts. If she responds to this by moaning, twisting, or playfully kicking you, her desire is skyrocketing. If she looks at you like a broken vending machine that just took her quarter, then it's time to give it up and dish it out.

However, even if playful withholding doesn't work for everyone, the linear, standard modus operandi is a universal turnoff. If you are being playful and spontaneous, your partner will feel it. If you are going through the motions and not really applying your creativity, your partner will feel that too. The number one ground rule for oral sex, then, is to *enjoy* it. Play around enough to find out what your lover likes (and doesn't like!).

You can start from above or below—whatever you do, just avoid diving right in. From below tends to make a racier mood, while from above is more traditional and romantic. If you start from the top, kiss her neck, her breasts, and her stomach, slowly working your way down her torso. The breasts remain a major pit stop on the road to oral love. As desire heats up, you can continue caressing the breasts with your hands, but keep moving your lips in the direction of the vulva. Kissing the breasts can get things rather offtrack, which might be fun, but may also erode the patience you'll need for oral sex.

As you work your way down, spreading kisses, tongue tickles, and little gentle bites, use your hands to stroke your way past the hips and to the inner thigh and knee area. Stroke and caress her legs, then start moving back in. Keep the kissing, caressing, and nibbling on high until you reach the very edge of the vagina. Kiss your way up and down one thigh, and then, just before you dive in, skip to the other inner thigh and start working your way out again.

Circling the vagina is key: it will heighten her sensations and get her fully aroused before you actually take the plunge. Do this a few times, but not more than three or four. When you're ready to go to it, get right up next to the vagina in the little cranny between the outside of the vagina and the thigh. Nibble her up. Brush your lips through the pubic hair (a soft, light sensation for her) and repeat on the other side. Light little bites are especially pleasurable in this area. On most women the skin here is sensitive enough to react strongly to the lightest touch, but not sensitive enough to feel pain.

At this point, she should be teased to the brink of a hissy fit won-

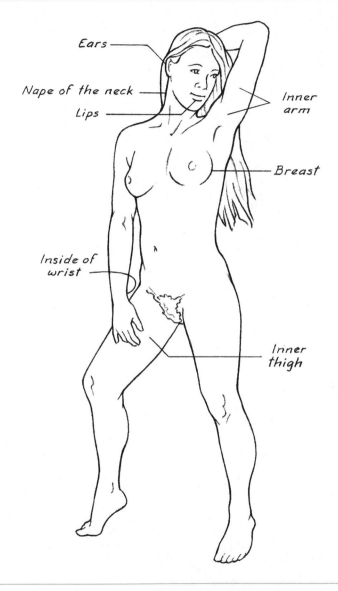

Ears

Nape of the neck

Lips

Inner arm

Breast

Inside of wrist

Inner thigh

All-over Erogenous Zones

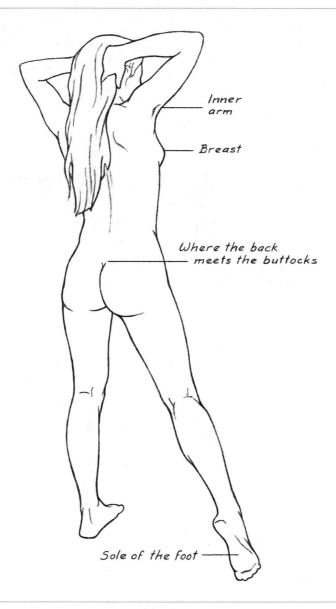

Inner arm

Breast

Where the back meets the buttocks

Sole of the foot

All-over Erogenous Zones

dering when you're going to finally make your move. Once she starts moaning, kicking you like a jockey riding a slowpoke, or trying to pull you closer to her, *c'est l'heure*. She's *prêt à manger*.

A great way to start is by taking the entire outer lips into your mouth in a big sucking, tugging kiss, or giving a wide-tongued, generous lick up the inside of each labia majora. These large, broad licks prepare the region to be stimulated, so spread the love. After you've prepped these lucky lips, skip right to the labia minora, which are much more sensitive. You can ask her to spread her lips for you, or you can spread them yourself.

L'entrée

Your first contact with the inner vagina must be excruciatingly slow and thick-tongued. Giving broad, long strokes to the inside of the labia, tell her she tastes good (if she does). If she doesn't, pull the game playfully into the shower, finger her until she comes prolifically, or just pop a breath mint in your mouth—which will also heighten her sensation. Whichever road you take, a long "mmm" once you're in the dugout will let her know you're having fun, and sends a few good vibrations up clitoris way.

The Lollipop Lick

Remember those gigantic swirling lollipops you had as a kid? Shoot for a similar surface area. Start at the perineum, and take it all the way up to the tip of the clitoral hood. Make your tongue as wide and flat as possible, and do at least seven (but not more than twelve) of these big, slow inner-lip lollipop licks. Start from bottom to top, because excitement will build as you near the clitoris, but trick her with a brush-by and a slow ensuing downward lollipop. And I mean *slow*, like five full seconds per lip-lick. You want to devour every inch.

This is a terrific time to check out the territory and see what kind of girl you've got under you. If she twists or moans when you're close to the vaginal canal, she may be waiting for penetration. If she gets hot or squeals when you pass over her clit, there's your jackpot. If she moans when you start the lick at the perineum, she might like anal stimulation. Just observe the signs and make a mental note.

Tongue Penetration

It appears that many men miss the point of tongue penetration altogether. If a part of my body is bigger, badder, and explicitly designed for penetration, why should I waste my time and exert so much energy just for a few tongueful inches? If the astounding benefits of tongue penetration aren't immediately apparent to you, keep the following things in mind.

Only about one-third of women can orgasm from intercourse alone. On the other hand, clitoral stimulation alone can give around two-thirds of women a nice big cookie. But even when tongue penetration alone misses the point, it's still an incredibly pleasurable sensation. There are a couple of reasons why women like it when the tongue is used to penetrate the vaginal canal. First, you can press the taste bud side of your tongue to the top of the vaginal wall, and if you tilt her hips forward enough, or use a position that helps out with oral penetration, you might be able to make good on her G-spot. Second, you can point and narrow your tongue and very lightly and rapidly dart it back and forth in a motion that will drive her wild. These fleeting, tantalizing sensations will primarily make her hungry for more. You needn't try to make her climax this way. However, you can get her to climax through tongue penetration alone if you incorporate another move.

To add the ultimate kick, and make tongue penetration rival the real thing, suck the entire labia minora and the clitoral hood into your lips before you insert your tongue. (You can alternate with your fingers if your tongue gets tired—though after all the exercises you've done there's no reason why it should.) As you point and insert your tongue, begin to dart it back and forth, simulating intercourse. Now allow the edge of your lip to rub back and forth over her clit hood—after all, you have it right there under your lip, you might as well make the most of it. In time with your tongue, plunge over it again and again, with a little more intensity and suction each time, until she's turning to mush. Grabbing her buttocks and tilting her hips forward a little will do three things at once: give you better access for deeper penetration, create some breathing room for your nose, and give her a nice sensation on her ass. If you want to give her the tongue penetration to end all tongue penetrations, use your finger at this point to lightly stimulate her anus and perineum.

EXTRA AVENUES OF SEXPLORATION

Clitoral Stimulation

If your lollipop licks didn't reveal one specific area of sensitivity, you can go to work on the clit first. First approach the clit from the outside of the labia. The clitoris is most easily stimulated by a light, rolling motion with the (well-lubed, short-nailed) fingertip.

Many people seem to believe that the simple act of licking a clitoris with the tongue should be enough to rocket their partner into outer space. This is rarely the case. Instead, alternate your licking with a gentle rub with your fingertip. The fact that the clitoris is hooded results in the underside being extremely sensitive, while when the lips are pulled back the exposed tip is hypersensitive. You have to follow *her* on this one, because most women prefer one place or the other.

Sweeping the Clitchen Floor

When you're ready, use your tongue and lips to exert pressure in the general area, using your tongue to stroke upward from the entrance of the vagina to the top of the hood. You should be able to feel the clit resisting your pressure. You can simply use the first third of your tongue to make a repetitive sweeping motion up and over the clitoral hood, varying your pressure until you strike some gold. Make sure that you begin from just below the clit, and that the tip of your tongue is curled up enough to reach the underside of the hood.

Suck It Up

As if you were eating a bonbon, suck and nibble the clit through the labia, or for a more sensitive woman, begin your lingual caresses at the bottom of the clitoris and work it gently back and forth while noting her responses. When you get some soft moans, push the labia away with your upper lip, point your tongue, and stroke her clit's underside with a moist tip at a medium-fast stroke.

- If you do not keep the area moist at all times, these sensations may change from pleasing to painful.

- Sucking like a Hoover will desensitize the area—the light touch is your best friend here.

- Your tongue is not a piston—more subtle strokes are necessary.

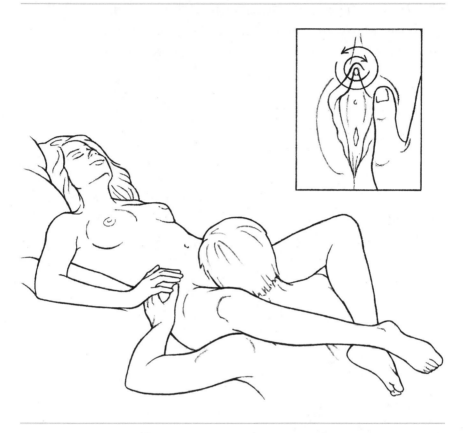

Lick Her Clit, Alternating Licks with Light Finger Touches

Clitnapping

When the sighs start getting longer and more intense, you can give stronger strokes. Keep using your fingers or lips to hold the labia back from the clit. Returning to a slightly more gentle and broad-tongued stroke, introduce your tongue directly to the top of the clit. When your girl gives you a sigh like the introduction is going well, point the tip of your tongue more and stroke the clit aggressively. If this is met with more sighs of glee, you can close your lips on the clit and suck it entirely into your mouth. Once there, squeeze it with your lips, tickle the thing wild with the pointed tip of your tongue, and give it

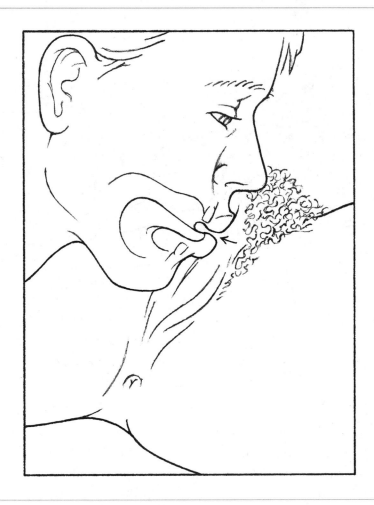

Take the Clit Gently Between Your Lips

an absolute lashing with aggressive, wild strokes (but don't use your teeth!). Or, you can just bring it into your mouth (itself a pleasurable sensation) over and over, using a rolling motion of the lips. If she convulses, slow down and lighten up; if she yells or moans, bring it on. Fireworks should be imminent.

If fireworks were not imminent, don't be disheartened. Some clits need heavy-duty treatment. Think of this as an excellent opportunity to truly distinguish yourself as a fabulous oral lover. With a less reactive clit, you can be much more experimental and creative, while a supersensitive one has to be handled with care.

The Viscous Twirl

The first thing to do with an unresponsive clit is to relax. You are much bigger and smarter than this pea-size love button. Separate the clit completely from the vaginal lips and isolate it entirely. No distractions. Now suck it up into your mouth, keeping it erect by creating an airtight vacuum with your lips. Give a nice aggressive flick directly on the clit. This has a much more intense effect on a vacuumed clit. Then, depending on your girl's response, switch to some teasing swirls, which will be much more intense inside your mouth than on a clit that's free to roam and get lost behind the labias. These swirls are best created by using the edge of the tongue to circle around and around the entire clit. Try both clockwise and counterclockwise— most women have a preference.

The Muhammad Ali

If she seems okay with the Viscous Twirl, keep the clit in your airtight (but not crushing) vacuum and give the clit a rapid, back-and-forth licking. Fly like a butterfly and sting like a bee. If she starts to convulse, intersperse these aggressive strokes with the soft, long twirls, and then return, switching to light flicks with just the tip of your tongue, slowly getting heavier and faster until you've got her number.

The Light Flick

You can give a strong but light flick particularly suited for the airtight vacuum by pointing your tongue, pulling it back into your mouth cavity, and making sure that even though the clit is clitnapped into your vacuum, your tongue has plenty of room to maneuver. Try both up-and-down and side-to-side light flicks, because again, the clit is a finicky customer and will respond very differently to minute changes in what you're serving. These light flicks are also excellent for anal stimulation.

Lend That Helping Hand

Just because you've vacuumed up the pleasure bud, don't forget about the rest of your lady. Hold her body with your hands, grabbing and massaging her flanks. In certain positions, you can also caress her breasts. Holding on to her will also give you the pleasure of feeling orgasms roll through her body. Also, just because you have engaged the clit, doesn't mean you have to stay there. Intersperse your clit time with tongue penetration, anal play, generous G-spot fingering, and nibbles and licks everywhere. No reason to get too single-minded—it's supposed to be fun, after all.

Climbing Mt. Climax

When you're ready to initiate a climax, pull the clit back into the air-tight mouth vacuum and give a straight-up series of up-and-down strokes interspersed with side-to-side ones. You can change direction, but do not change the rhythm. If this is too much for her, place your tongue beneath her clitoris in your mouth and stroke it from below, which will create a slightly less intense sensation. If even this is too much for her, you can simply tap the clit in a rhythmic way, or gently oscillate your tongue from side to side in your mouth along the bottom of the clit.

Once you hear her breathing getting heavier and her inner thighs start to tremble, you've got your winning combination. Stay with this combination—don't change a thing. Whatever it takes—use a metronome if you have to—but keep that rhythm steady once she's on her way to the Big O. (If you won the lotto, you wouldn't suddenly change the numbers, right? Same deal.)

The Delicious Aftermath

When she's had an orgasm, don't stop. Maybe men have orgasms like a big firecracker; women are like roman candles. So keep going long enough to determine whether another set is coming. Don't worry—she'll let you know when she's had enough. And if you've performed all the exercises in this book, you'll be able to explore those limits with her.

Once it's over, her vagina will be very sensitive. She may suddenly push your face away—don't be offended by this. It simply means that the area has become so sensitive that further stimulation would be painful. When this threshold isn't quite reached, some oral sex lovers like to stay after the orgasm, making their tongues long and wide, and laying them over the vagina like a big warm cover. This is fine, but make sure you don't move. After a couple of minutes, you can raise your head and feel the wind on your face. If she's motionless, you've done a good job.

Don't Diss the Postcoital Kiss

Remember that oral sex can be performed both before and after penetration. If you are a man performing oral sex on a woman, be aware that there is nothing in nature other than your own fund of energy to stop you from performing oral sex on your woman after intercourse. It feels really great and can lead to multiple orgasms, so don't automatically rule it out. Many men find the idea of taking their own semen into their mouth a turnoff. This is the definition of a culturally learned attitude. That stuff's good for you—filled to the brim with vitamins and nutrients. If you really can't get over it, hop in the shower with your lady of choice, but recognize that your squeamishness is unnecessary.

THINK OUTSIDE THE "BOX"

It seems appropriate to mention here that there are spots all over the body that enjoy caresses and stimulation, not just the vagina. The breasts, the arms (especially the sensitive skin toward the armpits), the neck, the earlobes and behind the ear, as well as the thighs and lower back, all deserve their share of stimulation. So it is with the anus. If we're just talking nerve endings, the anus is the only spot on the body that even begins to rival the clitoris. When you're comfortable with the idea of rimming (or anal play), you unlock new portals to pleasure for yourself and others. Remember, there is plenty of plastic wrap in this world to keep you covered. (And if you're high on style with the cash to prove it, you can actually buy the dental dams.) "Oral sex" does not have to be vagina-specific or vagina-limited. Erotic sensations can be produced in many places and can create orgasms that rival or put to shame vagina-centered ones.

Before any sexual act, you and your partner should both be scrupu-lously clean, which is one reason why showering together beforehand is such a wonderful idea. For anal oral sex (anilingus), cleanliness is a must and I recommend a shower and a dental dam. But do whatever you need to. This is worth it.

If your partner is open to this idea, it is best for her to be on all fours with her head and shoulders tilted down and perhaps resting on a pil-low. Approach her from above in order to ensure maximum access to the anal region.

Point your tongue—though you are not going to penetrate her, your attempt to do so will create marvelous sensations. If your part-ner is responsive to this—which she may not be, because of personal discomfort or the cultural stigmas attached—you will have yet another way to provide her with profound pleasure.

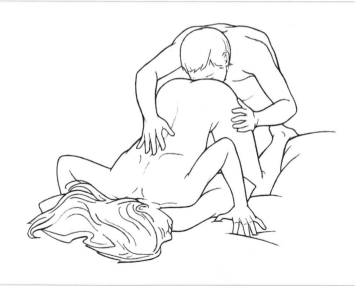

Anal Stimulation: Thinking Outside the "Box"

Anyone who judiciously applies the techniques outlined in this chapter can make themselves an expert at oral sex. As in real estate, the trick to much oral sex is "location, location, location." But these are merely the basics of that cunning kiss, cunnilingus.

12

Put Some Ambition in Your Position:
Postures That Will Make Her Purr

HOOSE YOUR POSITIONS wisely, because you're probably going to be asked for repeat performances. Remember that if something sounds like it might be too strenuous for you, you're probably right. The best positions are more about precision than brute strength, though there's something to be said for being daring.

Here are a few primers to get you ready for the more advanced techniques.

START YOUR ENGINES

The Most Comfortable Position Ever
Though we'll go into more advanced positions later, one of the most comfortable may be for your woman to lie across the bed, her legs hanging to the floor. Kneel on the floor (maybe with a towel or pillow under your knees to maximize comfort) and bring her hips to where you have good access to the full vagina. In this way, you can provide her with a wide range of sensation, and your flexibility of

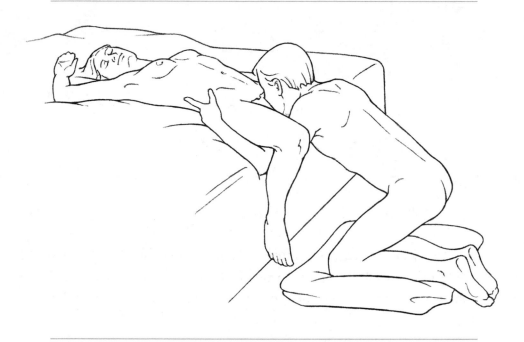

The Most Comfortable Position Ever

movement will keep you comfortable and creative without the tension on your back and neck muscles that would result from attempting the same feats flat on the bed.

Once you've developed your oral skills so that you are not easily thrown off by the positioning of your body, it is time to experiment with other positions.

Flapping Legs

This position is essentially the basic comfortable position recommended in the first part of this section, only the person giving oral sex is further up on the bed. This creates a little more strain in the back and neck muscles, but it's worth the trouble because the angling of the woman's legs will create better access to the clitoris and deeper penetration possibilities. The woman's legs are bent, with her feet resting on her lover's shoulders. Her pelvis is curved much more upward than

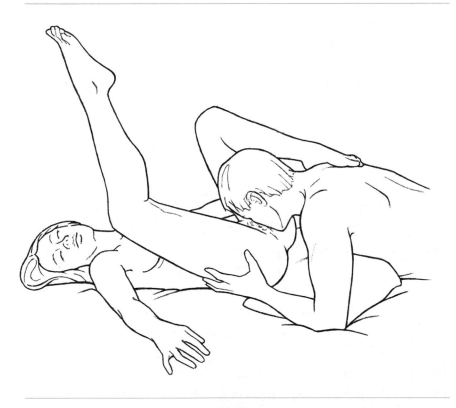

Flapping Legs

in the first position, and one leg may even be resting down her partner's back. To create more access as needed, you can edge your shoulders upward and press her thighs back further. This is a great position for incorporating a little vibrator or anal play. As she approaches climax, she will alternately press down on your shoulders with the pads of her feet and flap them in the air. This position provides great access for upward strokes, and you can angle your arms a little under her body for support.

Captured Tortoise

For superior access (but less flapping), try Captured Tortoise. In this, the woman holds her legs to her chest, providing you with total access. This is a great position if your woman is into penetration—combining a vibrator or dildo with your oral stimulation is a godsend here. Be careful, because as she gets excited her body may twist and, because she is holding her legs to her chest, she may flip over. Stabilize her by helping her hold one leg with your arm (but not too hard).

A Word on 69s

Sixty-nining basically involves simultaneous oral sex. This has always seemed more like a novelty act to me than a genuine source of erotic satisfaction, since the ability to give oral sex is very much compromised by the mutual stimulation. However, it still seems to be the rage, so someone out there must think it's hot stuff. The position most often used in 69s has two variations.

In the first, the woman is on her back, her knees raised and spread, with her partner above her, poised so that by bringing bodies together both partners can reach all the lucky parts to receive stimulation. In the second position, the partners switch places. Technically speaking, it can be performed side to side, but this can get clunky because too

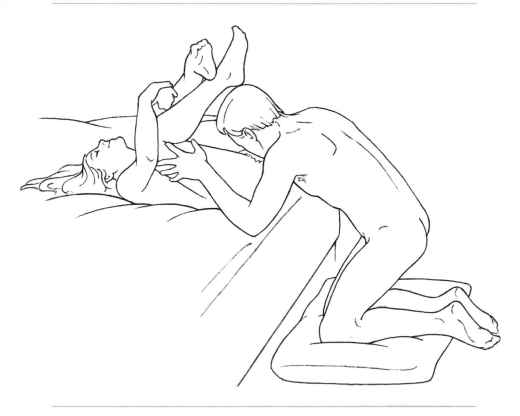

Captured Tortoise

many legs have to be suspended in the air. If you want to try it, cradle your head in the inner part of her thigh and make sure your hips are adequately thrust forward.

The 69 is a practice of great antiquity and can be quite fun, but proper oral sex can rarely be performed during it.

Ball and Sock It

If your lady is more sensitive on the left or right side of her clitoris, switch up the Captured Tortoise with the Ball and Sock It. (And yes, you are the ball.) Your partner should lie on her back, with one leg extended and one bent at the knee for maximum access. Come at her from an angle, straddling the extended leg. Give her circular strokes and find that sensitive spot on the right or left side of her clitoris.

The Pleasure Plank

Some people like the sensation of having their legs together during oral sex. This position can be a great teaser when you are initially working your way down. Holding her just above the hips with your hands and straddling her closed, extended legs, come at her clitoris from the top of her vagina.

Some women have a hypersensitive clit, and this position gives them painless pleasure by buffering the vibrations from your tongue. Of course, if you've done the exercises in this book, you should be able to give feathery strokes of infinite lightness, but otherwise this position can be a fun way to pick up some of the slack or to tease her as a prelude to something more.

The 6

Another slack picker-upper is the 6. This is essentially a 69 position with you on top, but your body is off to the side and she is just relaxing. Coming at her from above, this position is a relief for your head and neck muscles, and is great for a woman who loves a downward stroke.

However, if you use the position we initially recommended, where you are on the floor and she is on the bed, and you have relaxed your neck, throat, and head muscles with the tensing and relaxing exercises

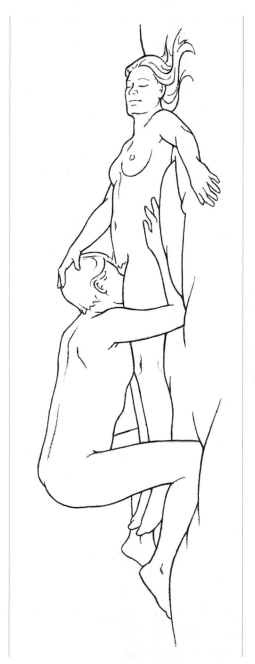

The Pleasure Plank

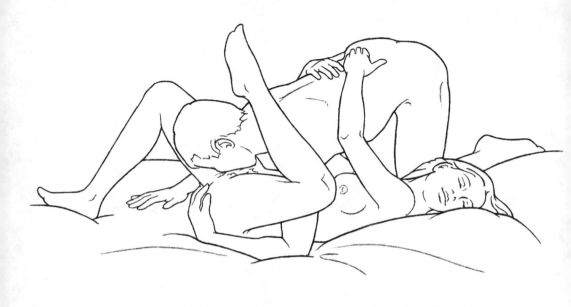

The 6

in chapter 9, you will never experience a need for this position except perhaps as a way to change things up.

The Yoga Payoff

Lying on her back, let your partner use her feet and legs to hoist herself up your kneeling body. Her weight should be resting on her shoulders, not her neck. From this angle, you can get a great view during oral sex—and this is a particularly nice position if your woman has a fabulous pair of breasts. Have fun watching her experience all of the erotic sensations she's feeling as you go to town on her clitoris. Don't bother with oral penetration or G-spot stimulation from this

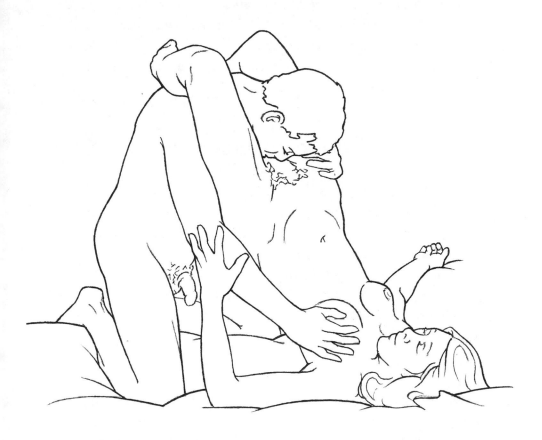

The Yoga Payoff

position. The combination of clit-nuzzling and the breast caresses you can give are the main attraction. Make sure to give your lady plenty of support in this one.

You may want to try all of these positions as you discover the areas where your partner is most sensitive. If you are having trouble in any of these positions, lightly changing the angle of the legs, placing one over your shoulder, or shifting the weight in your torso will help you get to that perfect spot.

POSITIONS FOR ORAL PENETRATION

Unlike during coitus, the vagina does not get its fair share of game during oral sex. This is because most people have not figured out how to insert their tongue far enough (and skillfully enough) into the vagina to reach the points of sensitivity that provide the hottest sensations of pleasure. Most of the positions that make this possible require a level of athleticism difficult to find in modern-day America. (I'm not sure where you *could* find it, but I'd be happy to go there.) So instead, what you can do is this:

The Boston Crab
Have your partner arch her back sharply on the bed (some supporting pillows here are nice) so that her body is very nearly in the position wrestlers call the Boston Crab. From a kneeling position on the floor, this will give you the maximum penetration possible. Remember that the vagina is cleaner than your mouth, and be bold.

The areas of sensitivity in the vagina typically have to be developed for them to be responsive to stimulation. The sensitive areas occur where the pubococcygeus muscle attaches at the bottom of the vagina to support it.

These points are as rich in nerve endings as Texas is in oil, so dig

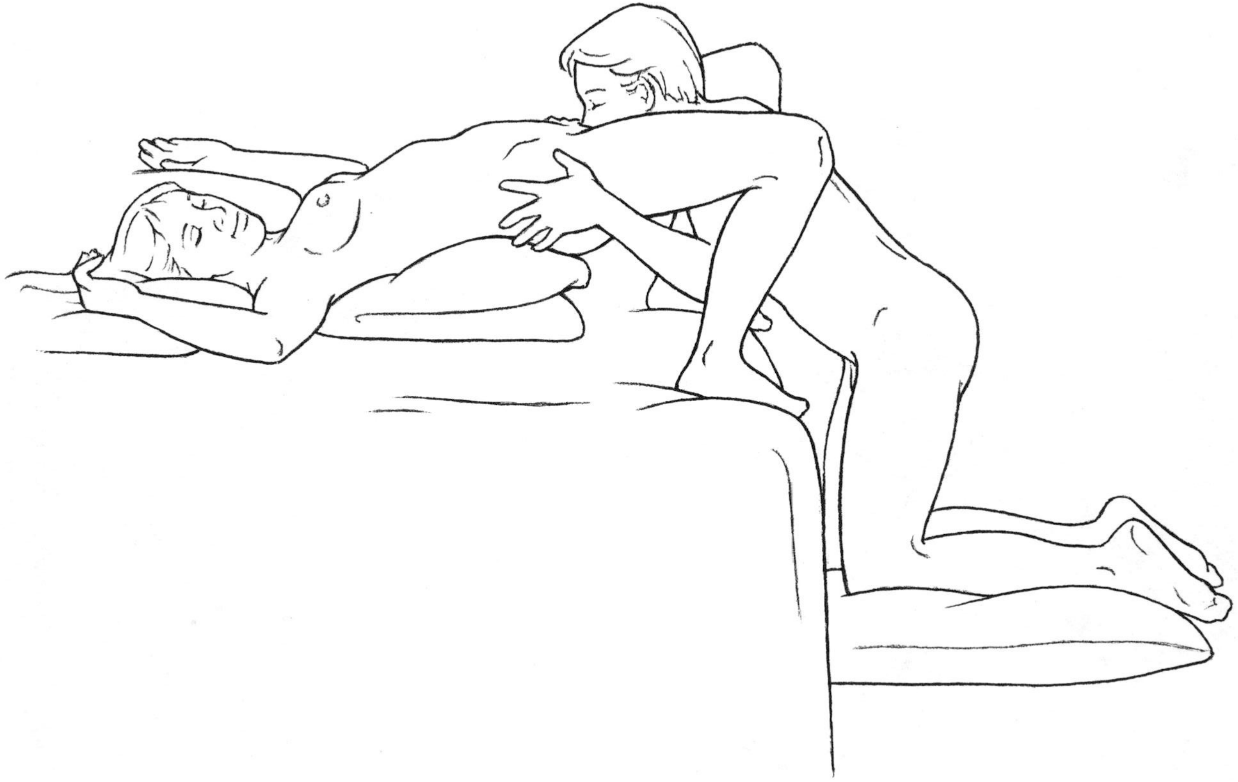

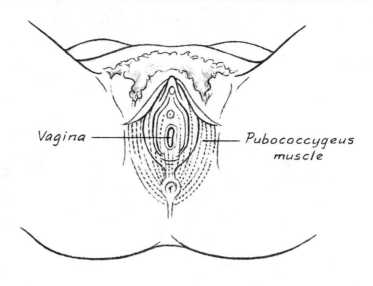

Vagina ——————— ——————— Pubococcygeus
                                    muscle

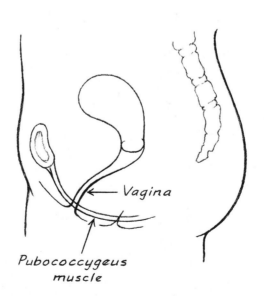

Vagina

Pubococcygeus
muscle

Locating the Pubococcygeus Muscle

in. The main issue here is your partner's comfort—the Boston Crab doesn't sound fun, and it isn't. But if she has learned to react to this area, she'll be duly motivated to hold her position for as long as humanly possible. And if you can roll your tongue, for god's sake do it now.

Once you've found the spots, slide your tongue in and out as if you were having sex, while making sure that the tip of your tongue caresses the areas where the muscle connects to her vagina. There is nothing in the vagina to tell you where these muscles attach, so you will have to study the diagram and make an educated guess. But you'll know it when you've found them. The neighbors might, too.

Remember that women are sensitive all over their bodies, and their pleasure will likely follow your tongue wherever it strays. Do not stress about these spots—they are simply special benefits to oral sex that you might be lucky enough to bump into. But you can give deeply satisfying oral sex—even hair-pulling, mercy-yelling, nail-sinking oral sex—without ever engaging them. So don't stress about it.

Brunch

This is a great position for a woman who likes to be on top. Lie down somewhere that elevates your head and has something for her to hold on to. If you have a bed with a frame, the headboard usually works best because you can support your head and neck with pillows. Have her come from above and essentially squat over your face. The visuals of her breasts will be worth the forfeiture of control. She will probably rub her vagina more deeply into your mouth than you are accustomed to—take this as an opportunity to learn exactly what she likes and when, because when she's ready for lighter strokes she'll pull up and forward.

This is a great moment to use your hands to grab her buttocks, stroke her lower back, and run your fingers up and down her chest and body. Plus, when she arches her back gently in response to the tingling sensations of pleasure, the visuals of her breasts will get even better.

Brunch for the Self-Stimulator

Fun twists (some literal) on brunching positions are only as limited as your imagination. If you'd like to give yourself a little hand job while brunching, have her assume the same position on a sofa, with her knees on the edge and hands on the back of the sofa. You can sit with your back against the sofa and lean your head back until it's comfortably resting beneath her. Have her lean down until the positioning is right, and go for it. The added extension of her body makes this position especially fun for anal play. You lose the breast visuals in this one, but if you're ready for a little self-stimulation, the trade-off is a good one.

Brunch for the Naughty Patient

Another great position for brunch that's sure to drive her wild involves you resting on a bed (or sofa) with your head hanging off the edge (or the raised arm). Have her stand up over your head, and make sure there is some room on either side because when things heat up, she is going to reflexively want to place a hand down for support. Have her spread her legs just enough for good access. This is a wonderful position for a woman who favors downward strokes, and a special position for you because you can easily incorporate both hands to further stimulate her clit and other sensitive spots. For a woman who likes anal stimulation, this position allows you to create diverse sensations with your tongue tickling her backside while your fingers can drive her into orbit. Because at least one of her hands are free, she can show you exactly how she likes to be rubbed.

POSITIONS FOR PORNO WATCHING

If your lady is turned on by visual stimuli, allow her the pleasure of multiple flicks. Some heterosexual women like all-female porn, while others like hetero and even all-male porn. Never judge a partner based on the kind of porn they like. It doesn't necessarily mean anything about their actual sexual preferences. However, you should never watch anything that makes you uncomfortable. Remember that videos are supposed to be fun and are meant to stimulate the imagination. So hold the gavel for now.

Sofa Porno

The most comfortable porno position is probably the Sofa. Have her sit on one arm of the sofa facing the screen, spreading her knees wide and edging herself forward to the edge of the cushion. Her arms on the back of the cushion will be an important source of stability in this position. You can sit on the sofa in a doggie-style position, resting on your knees and elbows. Arching your back will add to her visuals. She may grab your head or hair with one hand and press you more deeply into her. This is a natural response to this position, and if it makes you uncomfortable, feel free to simply nudge her hand away. If she strokes your head and hair however, the presence of her hand here can be quite delightful.

Armchair Porno

This position is for the hard-core porn–loving woman. You'll want to bring a pillow along for your knees. Have her sit in a chair with her buttocks supported by enough pillows to angle her hips upward, and make sure she is close enough to the edge of the chair for you to get access to the key players. Sitting on the floor or on your knees (this depends on the height of the chair), you can use your tongue to stim-ulate her clit and your hands for simultaneous penetration.

Because there is little physical contact between your bodies, you may want to heighten the tease of this position by kissing her all over her legs and thighs while the porno is beginning, and circling the prey a little until she's positively drooling for you.

There are too many positions to include them all, but these basic in-gredients should give you enough elements to begin mixing it up on your own. Remember that the only bad oral sex is boring oral sex, and as long as you stay out of the shower the likelihood of bodily in-jury is fairly low.

13

Vibrators, Dildos,
and Other Miscellany for Misbehaving

- Rule One: Don't knock sex toys until you've seen what they can do.
- Rule Two: Always, always, always wash your sex toys.

VIBRATORS

Let's start with the introductory vibrator, the kind you can buy in many sex shops; it's about four inches long and requires an AA battery. Many women like to travel with these because they are discreet—and powerful. Sometimes they come with a penis-replica plastic sleeve, which makes it more of a dildo (which is a penis replica made of plastic or sometimes glass, while a vibrator contains batteries and, well, vibrates). Do not be afraid of this item. This is going to be a good friend of yours, and never make your woman choose between her vibrating dildo and you. You may not like the choice she makes.

This device can be used to rocket oral sex into the next stratosphere. Gently insert it into the vaginal canal while you are licking and sucking the clitoris. As you establish a rhythm, feel free to begin rhythmically penetrating your woman with the vibrator. If you have the vibrator turned on, don't pump up the volume just yet. Instead, use long and deep, penetrating strokes interspersed with short, rapid strokes, depending on your mutual mood.

Some women like having the vibrator inserted as far as it will go, motionless but turned on, during oral sex so that they are receiving dual stimulation but are not overstimulated. These climaxes can be overwhelming anyway and are deeply rewarding—she may tightly grab you at the moment of climax and urge you to press the vibrator even more deeply into her. Do not be afraid of the climax-clutch. It is simply an expression of your woman's lasting excitement. When her climax is finished, she will probably push your face away and at this time you should gently, slowly remove the vibrator as well.

A related method involves inserting a very small vibrator in the anus. For the anally erotic gal, this is a real treat. A small vibrator can be slipped in during cunnilingus to excite and gratify. However, if you do not know the woman very well, or don't know her feelings about anal penetration, make sure she okays the move first.

You should never insert something into the anus as a "surprise" move. In order to insert anything into the anus, you need the conscious (but not overly, as in self-conscious) participation of your partner. You don't have to stop licking and caressing her—just cover it in a water-based lubricant like K-Y jelly and make sure she knows that its coming by gently circling the anus and tapping against it before you slip the vibrator in.

When you use the vibrator in the anus and your tongue and mouth on the clitoris, your woman will probably loose her cookies early on. But this is a fun alternative to the standard fare, and comes highly recommended.

If you and your partner are ready for another variation, try using a second vibrator. One vibrator is gently inserted into the anus in the manner described above, while the other (usually larger) vibrator is inserted into the vagina. A pulsing sensation will occur all over the woman's body when both vibrators are turned on and suddenly come into sync with each other. When the two vibrators, whose motors are not rotating at exactly the same speed, periodically drop into perfect phase with each other, the presence of you sucking and licking her clitoris becomes intensely pleasurable.

This isn't for everyday sex, but it is a wonderful way to spice things up and give her the kind of mind-blowing pleasure we all crave every once in a while.

DILDOS

The only thing as remarkable as the long history of the dildo (quite possibly the oldest sex toy on earth) is the variety of shapes, sizes, textures, and colors this handy sex asset has assumed. Some of them are tapered enough to make them great for anal play, while others are curved for G-spot stimulation. But they can all add to your oral sex repertoire by keeping one sensitive area engaged while you're busy with another. For G-spot stimulation, make sure you get something with a well-defined bulbous head, in addition to the traditional curved shape.

Available in glass, metal, acrylic, silicone, and a nearly limitless variety of other materials, dildos can range in style from the incredibly detailed and realistic to the fantastically abstract and unearthly—it's all up to you and your woman. The important thing to remember is that, even if you might see fabric or leather or horsehair dildos available, the only truly safe ones are those that can be washed and disinfected—

like glass (with no chips), acrylic, metal-plated, and silicone. A particular and lovely trait of the glass dildo is that it can be placed under hot or cold running water for just a few minutes to contribute a new range of sensations to your partner. A great sidekick for a warm, lively little tongue.

Products in silicone, however, rightly deserve their reputation as god's gift to sex toys. Silicone is smooth, nonsticky, and simultaneously resilient and soft. It absorbs body heat rapidly, so just rubbing it between your hands can make it something of a treat to gently insert into the orifice of your choice. Start playing with this stuff and you'll both be late to work for a week.

If you want to save some money, the products being made out of jelly aren't bad. Some people even prefer jelly to silicone (though I can't say I agree), and it's extremely inexpensive. The jelly starts to become opaque over time and also gets sticky just sitting around (eventually looking like an old lollipop).

Like all sex toys, dildos should be washed after every use, but the jelly products in particular pick up bits of dust and hair floating around everyday, so you should give them a nice washing both before and after. The final note on jelly toys is that they will always smell like plastic—like when a "made in China" product is first taken out of its airtight wrapping. This smell never completely leaves the jelly sex toy, though it lessens somewhat. So, if your nostrils don't flare with pleasure at the idea, stick to silicone.

ANAL PROBES

And you thought you had to be abducted by aliens first. Anal probing feels much more pleasurable than it sounds (though, as with all acquired tastes, it starts to sound as good as it feels) and lots of time and energy have been spent creating products that maximize this pleasure.

A metal or acrylic dildo is fine for vaginal play, but something softer and more forgiving is required for the anus. When selecting a probe, make sure you get something soft enough, and with a graduated shaft that will allow you to insert to the desired width. Also, make sure you get something with a nicely sized handle. You don't want to lose your grip—and neither does your partner. As indicated by its name, the probe is longer than other toys created for anal insertion and is a great way to find out exactly where your woman wants anal stimulation. Be aware that probes require constant attention as they tend to shift more than plugs.

ANAL PLUGS

Anal plugs are endlessly fun—so endless, in fact, that some people start wearing them all the time. (That doesn't necessarily mean I'm one of them.) They come with a gorgeous array of decorations, using gemstones and different designs to give the butt a fashionable, naughty, or bejeweled look when inserted. The most important thing to remember when selecting an anal plug—as with all anal toys—is the size. A true beginner should start with something under seven ounces, no longer than two inches, and no wider than 1¼ inch at its widest point. If this is your first time, go for something nicely tapered for an easier entry, with a well-flared base so that it won't slide too far in. If you plan to start wearing one all the time, just make sure yours has a very long, narrow (one inch or less) neck to keep it from falling out. That might be rather difficult to explain at a morning meeting.

ANAL BEADS

"I'll wear my pearls." Ever wonder how strands of beads became so popular? Sadly, it has nothing to do with the fact that they're such awesome sex toys. This toy is a great introduction to anal play, and usually consists of beads graduated in size from a few eighths of an inch in diameter on up. (Selecting a strand that ranges from three-eighths to one inch will provide a little something for everyone.) Also, make sure that the beads are made of a smooth material. Metal beads are to be avoided, as is any material harder than your finger.

Insert the beads gently, one bead at a time, into your (forewarned) partner until you reach the bead that almost won't go in. At the moment of orgasm (or whenever you feel the time is right), pull the beads out in one long, continuous motion by the ring or handle. Some people go wild over the insertion, but most find that the boon of the beads lies in their sudden extrication (which can heighten orgasms considerably). A variant of the anal beads is an apparatus with a series of round, consecutively smaller spheres. This can be used similarly to an anal plug, but has some of the advantages of the beads. Also, as the beads commonly use nylon thread, this toy has the added benefit of being completely washable.

The most important ingredients when using sex toys, especially with anal toys, are lube and relaxation. If you choose toys that are smooth in texture, and don't fall for the "my eyes were bigger than my . . ." syndrome that hits all of us every once in a while, these toys will add hours—and perhaps a lifetime—of new pleasure to your repertoire. To keep your toys clean, consider using them with a condom, and use only water-based lube on or around them.

14

Techniques to Wake Up
the Neighborhood

Is sex dirty? Only if it's done right.
—WOODY ALLEN

UNTIL NOW, WE have dealt primarily with the essential or basic oral sex techniques. At this point, you are equipped with all the skills you need to become a master of the art. But if you want to truly drive your woman into *la folie*—mad fits of joy that can barely be described by any human language—try employing some of these more advanced techniques. Remember, every woman is different, so your best guide is always your partner. These are simply possible sources of pleasure for her.

MANY SOURCES, MANY PLEASURES

Remember that your woman is sensitive all over her body, and that you can always use your hands to bring her closer to you and touch more of her. A great way to heighten sensation is to begin sucking the clitoris gently and repetitively, much as a baby might nurse a nipple. Do not suck too hard—you don't want to hurt her or desensitize the area. Combine this gentle suction with a side-to-side motion of your head, so that different parts of your soft, full lips come into contact with her clitoris.

When she is heavily roused, but not yet orgasming, place your fingers in her vaginal canal and lubricate them with the moisture you find there. Or, you can use your own saliva. Now apply your lubricated finger to her anus, giving it a good covering (with or without a dental dam, as you two see fit). Once her anus is sufficiently lubricated to allow it, gently insert one finger there and one finger into

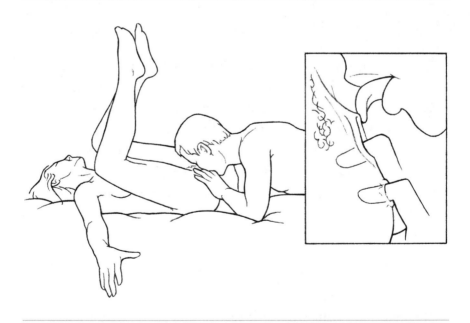

Multiple Stimulation

her vagina. This must be done extremely gently and slowly, caressingly. By this time, the woman is highly sensitive in the entire region, so make your fingers go as slowly as you possibly can. When your fingers are inserted, don't move them around. Just let them go in as far as seems comfortable for both of you and give circular, sucking motions on the clitoris, then begin to slowly increase your pace and pressure. If she's truly comfortable with it, the threefold intensity will drive your partner into wild, crazy bliss.

THE JACKHAMMER

If you have ever seen someone jackhammering on the street or sidewalk, perhaps you noticed how they plunge in for a few intense moments, then stop and stare at the hole they made, then plunge in again for another short duration. You, believe it or not, are going to take your cues from these guys to elicit major orgasms from your honey.

Begin performing cunnilingus on her with whatever technique she finds most pleasurable. It should be a position and method that allows both of you maximum comfort, because this technique takes longer than most (but also involves a lot of resting time for you). Give her whatever oral stimulation she wants until you have brought her just to the brink of climax. This is a point you should learn to recognize without her help as soon as possible, because if she can tell you that she's about to climax she's wrong. She shouldn't be able to speak at this point. For this technique to work you must bring her to the very cusp of orgasm.

Without tipping that delicate scale and letting everything release, when you see that she is about to climax, stop stimulating her and completely stop touching her body, remove your mouth and pull back a few feet from her vagina. This is orgasm deprivation, and it is going to increase the intensity of the orgasm she experiences very seriously. Wait like this for thirty-five seconds (count in your head), which is the amount of time it takes for her body to subside from its preorgasmic state. (I envy the participants of the study that discovered this fact.) Feel free to make intense eye contact and talk very dirty during this time. When the count is up, dive back in and bring her back to the cusp of orgasm. She will want to explode on contact, but as soon as she's back on the verge of orgasming, pull away again.

This time, count to fifteen, and once again begin your stimulation. Bring her body to the brink of implosion and pull back without touching her at all. Repeat this action one last time. She will most likely climax with the first contact of your tongue to her body, but this climax will be unlike others—the force and intensity of it will rival all that came before. Throbbing waves of pleasure will ride up and down her body, possibly down to her ankles and toes.

Each time you bring her to the cusp of climax without going over, you heighten the sensation of her ultimate climax. This mechanism works like one of those toy cars that you pull backward along the floor to rev up—the more times you pull it back without letting it go, the faster it goes when you do finally release it. But like the toy car, if you spend too much time revving, she might not go at all. That is why the timing and being able to read your lover's signs and signals are vital to this powerful technique. If you are not stealing her from just under the cusp of the orgasm, the intensity will not build and she will just get frustrated. If this starts to happen, just give her what she wants. "Kisses are a better fate than knowledge," as e. e. cummings said. Finding out about a technique is never more important than the experience of intimate pleasure together, so keep your priorities straight.

ORAL SEX FOR THE GOURMAND

The following substances can heighten the experience of oral sex for both of you. There are a couple of basic rules regarding how foods can be incorporated into your sexual play. The vagina is a delicate and often unpredictable creature, and tends toward infections and complications of all varieties. Therefore, to play it safe, if you place anything that contains oils (in many lubes), sugars (in many treats), or dairy products (including whipped cream from a can) into your woman, she will need to wash it out afterward with plenty of water and a nonirritating soap.

Also, if you're planning to use a condom later, make sure you don't put anything with sugar or oils in her. No matter how spanking clean you lick her—and we hope you're licking every last drop—sugar and oils can leave trace amounts that will eat little holes in your condom. And a hole-filled condom is no condom at all.

Never put anything in your woman that includes meat products or chemicals of any kind. This includes most household products, but since you probably have enough sense to avoid those anyway, keep in mind that this also includes soap. Sometimes guys sweetly offer to bathe their woman in the shower, which is a wonderful, wet sensation, but they take it too far when the bathing involves putting soap between the lips of the vagina. This creates an acidic, painful feeling and disturbs the pH levels of the vagina. Essential oils (including patchouli), mouthwash, and toothpaste are all verboten. If you want a minty fresh sensation, popping a breath mint will give her tingling, breezy sensations without hurting her. However, since most breath mints include sugar, she'll need to bathe afterward. Sugar-free breath mints are completely safe. Douches are bad for her, so even if you see one in a flavor you'd like, try to find something else with the same taste.

The most important thing to consider when selecting your oral sex menu, aside from her vagina's health and happiness, is the drip factor, because what goes in must come out.

Chocolate

The consistency of chocolate syrup is too thin to make the flavor very intense for oral sex, and it will ruin whatever fabric you're having fun on. Visually this is also somewhat disturbing. If you play with chocolate syrup in the bed at night, in the morning it'll look like a massacre took place. If you want to use chocolate, avoid the syrup and opt for a product with a thicker consistency such as Nutella, chocolate icing from a can, or a chocolate paste from the sex shop. (The Body Talk Chocolate Tattoo Kit actually tastes like gourmet chocolate, if you're a stickler for the good stuff like I am.) Because it's less runny, you'll be able to provide her with a wider variety of sensations while you eat it off, instead of simply chasing its rivers down her torso as they make their way to your sheets. The thicker consistency also makes for tons of fun with a paintbrush (à la *The Pillow Book*). Painting on your lover can be incredibly sexy, and it's even more fun when the paint is edible. Those sex-oriented "finger paints" they sell in sex shops, by the way, taste downright awful. It's fun to get all Jackson Pollock on your lover, but make sure you use something that's meant to be digested.

Honey

Honey is a safer and in many respects more satisfying choice, because it's usually on hand, but it's also hard to get out of fabrics and demands a shower afterward. (Unless, that is, you like the bizarre sound effects created by peeling your honey-pasted bodies apart.)

Ice

Ice is the only 100 percent safe and clean-up free sex food. Lightly and playfully stroking a chip of ice along the inner lips of the vagina can add a marvelous feeling. If you want to use ice, gently run a small ice cube up and down the labia majora. When this has tantalized, place it in your mouth and perform oral sex as you normally would. Try placing the ice behind your tongue, allowing the lips and vagina to warm, and then suddenly releasing the ice for only as long as it takes for her to squeal.

Lubes

Flavored lubes wear promising labels, but rarely live up to them. Some of them use evil sugars and oils, so read the ingredients. Water-based is always preferable, and don't be afraid to buy a few and taste-test. When you find one you like, the investment pays back in spades. Peppermint almost always holds up, and for good flavoring ID Juicy Lube can usually be counted on.

Warming Oils and Lubes

If you use a heating massage oil, keep it out of your woman's vagina. It will make her feel like her lower lips are burning off, and when you go down on her, you'll feel pretty molten as well. If you want to use a warming product, make sure it says "lubricant" loud and clear somewhere on the packaging before you smear it in private places. Most of the warming lubes need to be rubbed, massaged, blown on, or licked to activate their warming qualities. Hot Licks is warming without being overpowering and has good-tasting flavors.

Home Cooking

Perhaps the most fun is the mutual refrigerator raid because it feels transgressive, and it's fun to surreptitiously sneak into the kitchen for such undomesticated reasons. Again, absolutely avoid meat products; and, though you should feel free to use them, make sure she knows to wash after dairy products or anything with oils or sugars. Butter, cream, peanut butter, and milkshakes are lots of fun at first, but too filling for most people. You want to stuff your face with your lover, not get a full stomach and fall asleep.

Ice cream is excellent, especially on and around the breasts. Ripe fruits such as strawberries, blueberries, and raspberries are wonderful to squish, smear, and then gobble and lick up. Jams and jellies have the same general issues as honey, and look even more like a murder scene in the morning than chocolate syrup. (However, don't avoid it simply because of the scene it makes. Just use sheets you don't mind down-grading.)

You may find that having a "quiet" dinner at home can be much more exciting and adventuresome than a night out on the town.

GROUP SEX

Three's Company

Think of all the people who have ever told you that they participated in an orgy. Divide that number in half. Again. This is closer to the ac-tual number of people you know who have been in a more-than-foursome.

The number of people who participate in threesomes is much greater. Threesomes can breed jealousies and difficult situations, so if you're considering this option make sure that all the people involved are *truly* comfortable with one another and with what you're doing. Other people prefer to try to avoid the issues by having the third party be a stranger. This does not necessarily eliminate all the potential problems. Be sure to have an open discussion with your partner before embarking on a group sex experience.

Most of the techniques in this book are based on the notion of two people privately pleasuring each other. However, oral sex is center stage in a group sex situation. Many women will not choose to put themselves in this position, because there is very high cultural stigma surrounding it. Other women may just not like it. Even the woman who desires it may not have the opportunity to experiment in this way because it involves finding two sexy people with whom she feels comfortable and who also feel comfortable with each other. But just in case all the pieces of the puzzle ever come together . . .

The Female Threesome

If it's a female threesome, the best way to heighten the oral sex sensations of the woman who is being the object of the other two's attentions is to begin with one person licking and sucking her breasts and nipples, caressing her upper body, and lightly stroking the sensitive parts of the woman's torso, hairline, anything that feels good. This playful caressing should continue throughout the entire sex act, with lots of intimate kissing. It will heighten the sensations of oral sex tremendously, as if you put a magnifying lens over every single sensation.

When the woman who is being attended to seems very aroused by the first partner, a good technique is for the third woman to then introduce herself by kissing and caressing her, starting from the bottoms of her legs and working her way up to the inner thigh. This will make the woman who is the center of attention sing with pleasure, though she will be hungering to develop things with the first partner.

Threesomes are just as psychological as any other form of sex (which means that it's very psychological) and withholding has as much or more impact here as it usually does. Two women can kiss each other, making the third visually aroused, then suddenly lavish attention on her unremittingly. The delay will heighten her sensations in whichever areas get explored.

Also, keep in mind that the first woman to get kissed will usually want to culminate her experience with her first partner. This can be made more intense by this first partner playing a little coy, as if she would rather have the other woman go down. Then, after she has spent lots of time kissing and caressing the woman who is being eaten out, she can suddenly take over and introduce a vibrator or dildo to heighten the surprise effect even more. Another level of withholding here can make a woman go berserk, if, the moment she switches places, she acts as if she might not fully do her part, and simply lightly strokes the labia and licks only along the outside of the labia minora. Then, when the woman being caressed in this fashion is about to explode with frustration, she can surprise her partner with even more daring moves than her predecessor.

The best threesomes involve a certain level of complicity—or at least the ability to read each other's cues—between two of the women. Another element that makes threesomes exciting (besides withholding and surprise) is confusion. It's extremely titillating to have two women simultaneously pleasuring you and to be so enveloped in sensations that you lose your sense of exactly who is doing exactly what. Having one woman stimulate the clit orally while the other stimulates the anus, while an arm or two caresses the breasts and thighs, is a wonderful way to achieve this confusion.

Like this, the two partners can trade off until the woman who is being pleasured has had so many orgasms that everyone has lost count. Her sighs of satisfaction will typically be followed by a changing of places.

The goal here is to have rapid-fire orgasms so that there is time and energy for everyone to experience the spotlight of pleasure. When you enter your threesome, keep in mind that group sex takes a lot longer than one-on-one sex when it's done right.

Including a Man (or Two!)

If a man—or two—is participating, it is common for one man to begin giving the woman oral sex, while the other fondles and kisses her breasts and mouth. These have to be men who are very comfortable with each other and the act they are performing. When she is near—but not quite at—the first orgasm, the man below can start having intercourse with her in gentle, long, slow strokes while the other man keeps caressing her breasts and torso, then moves his hands toward the vulva and stimulates her manually from above.

When her partner in coitus is approaching orgasm, the man performing oral sex on her can move back up to her mouth, slowly stroking and caressing her, and be fellated to orgasm simultaneously with the other man.

Do not be afraid to ask your partner questions about this and other oral experiences—it's the only reliable way to learn, and the more you know about the nature of her sexual desires, the better you can satisfy them.

Conclusion

THE BIGGEST SURPRISE to oral sex is how much you are going to enjoy taking your partner to these extremes of pleasure. The greater the arousal you produce in them, the greater the arousal you are likely to feel. Oral sex—when performed by someone skilled and confident in their abilities—is a concrete example of the pleasure of giving. The greater the degree of delight you produce within your partner's body, the greater pleasure your own will be able to experience. Just witnessing the kinds of orgasms sparked and kindled by the exercises and techniques in this book is a fantastic experience. If you truly utilize what you have learned here, you may see women pulling their own (and your) hair, ripping pillows, sheets, their clothing and your T-shirt if you're wearing one, screaming a wide variety of words (some expletives), and closing their eyes to lose themselves in the sensations of pleasure that beckon them. Furthermore, after these orgasms the recipient tends to become quite giving in nature for at least several hours, and sometimes days. Do not abuse this indulgent attitude toward you, but feel free to enjoy it.

> Smile—It's the second best thing you can do with your lips.
>
> —ANONYMOUS

ABOUT THE AUTHORS

MARCY MICHAELS is a consulting speech pathologist/audiologist and educator with over twenty-five years' experience in her field. She has worked with a broad and diverse clientele, ranging from actors and broadcasters to international businessmen and children. She has four degrees in speech and biology, including a premed program at NYU, a BS in speech and communication arts from Adelphi University, an MS in speech pathology and audiology from Long Island University, and a postgraduate degree in speech education from St. John's University. She lives in New York City.

MARIE DESALLE attended the Sorbonne, then graduated from Sarah Lawrence College in New York with a BA in writing. Her interest in sex has manifested itself in photography, writing, and other artistic forms of self-expression. She lives in New York City.